Extreme Weight Loss Hypnosis For Women: Affirmations & Guided Meditations For Rapid Fat Burn, Mindfulness & Healthy Eating Habits + Overcoming Food Addiction (Hypnotic Gastric Band)

Table of Contents

Introduction:

Hypnotherapy is a method of treatment in which a hypnotist offers some suggestions to a person for a desirable behavioural change. It works when there is focused attention and an altered state of mind. A person under hypnosis may subconsciously absorb all the communication that a hypnotherapist does. The critical mind of a person is lower down through the workload of messages and the change occurs because hypnotic induction allows a person to accept the suggestions for change and able to alter the core beliefs that might limit helpful actions. Through this natural treatment method, research evidence recently boosts the effectiveness of hypnotherapy in managing headaches, pain during invasive dental and other surgical processes, managing anxiety, stress, low mood, confidence building, weight loss and much more.

Hypnosis and weight loss have been explored with the help of several clinical experiments. The efficacy of clinical hypnosis has been established for the assurance of fruitful outcomes for overall health. A variety of medical and mental health disorders are now dealt with with the help of different techniques that hypnosis proposed. Typically for weight loss, hypnosis has been shown improvement in self-control, seeking lower body mass and resolving one's emotional conflicts. Eating problems i.e. excessive or restricting are both harmful for proper weight and women tend to be the victim of eating disorders more often than men however body image shatters in both genders equally. One of the potential factors behind the development of unhealthy weight gain and relevant issues is emotional instability.

Other options to manage weight include surgical procedures and therapeutic interventions. Fasting, chakra balancing, aromatherapy, Tai Chi, nutritional therapy, endoscopic procedures, injections, exercise and yoga are some of the commonly heard solutions. These procedures are time taking, short-term relievers and temporary with greater costs for an average person. There are painful consequences sometimes and it is almost impossible to maintain the benefits from these methods in the long term. Years of follow-up and constant effort are required for ideal weight management. Moderate weight loss goals and slow achievement is always considered more stable than the fastest quick fix. The opposite alternative of all these discussed quick fixers is a form of hypnosis called gastric band hypnosis.

Gastric band hypnosis works directly on the human subconscious mind. The suggestions are given in a way that induces a belief that a tight gastric band is tied around the stomach. It is a traditional concept of surgery through the band at the upper part of the stomach that limits food intake and consumption on daily basis without any alternative thought. The physical band encouraged weight loss but came with undeniably uncontrollable complications. This leads to modern hypnosis to create the experience of the band in imagination. We are what we believe, once we believe that we can eat lesser and healthy.

To accompany weight loss, other techniques are as follows:

Neuro-linguistic programming (NLP) is an approach that elaborates the methodology of communication that directs human beings to take action through a source of their preferred representational learning style through which they speak and listen and perceive sensory information with the help of five senses. One of them is dominant for an individual. The metaphors, expressions and images, sounds, textures that people understand and learn through are some of the ways to integrate verbal communication in hypnotic suggestions. The NLP suggestions even work strongly when the hypnotic state is induced. This is not a directly observed method to bring change in someone but even more influential with access directly to the subconscious.

Affirmations are very frequently combined with hypnotic suggestions for behavioural change. These are positive statements customized to strengthen the beliefs about whatever we want to achieve in life. They work one by one and enable us to modify our action accordingly. Hypnotic inductions facilitate the path of these affirmations to the human mind where we realize our competencies and efficiency. The work that we do is mostly regulated by the beliefs that we affirm ourselves since childhood. The unfortunate bundle of them are irrational, counterproductive, negative and damaging. To compensate for the persistent loss, affirmations are sent through hypnosis and change becomes faster.

Meditations are stress-managing exercises. Meditation is a practice that silently makes the stress levels down to earth. The meditation provides the surface for other similar opportunities to explore. The opportunities positively influence the mind and body to open up for wellbeing. It is guided through meditations and mindfulness exercises that focus is the road to success. The focus is enhanced when hypnosis is induced. It is predicted that the hypnotic state along with meditations smoothly shifts the human being into a fitness-oriented mindset. The connection of mind and body is essential for mind and body psychotherapies to function.

Eating habits and lifestyle guidelines are usually recommended in the shape of hypnotic suggestions for relapse prevention and triggers management. There are some specific triggers emotional, cognitive or behavioural for people that can cause binge eating and unhealthy food picking which is a disaster for the acquired success in weight loss and fat burning journey.

The purpose of the selection of given series of hypnotic scripts is to create a sequential stepwise combination of short, easy to understand non-invasive, pain-free and long-term benefits with a gastric band and complementary hypnotic scripts. Consider this book as an outline of natural remedies for your lifetime recovery from unpleasant body and weight-related issues. Always track the changes in your weight, emotions and another daily life routine between each script that you listen to every 3-4 days a week. Then compare these notes for your awareness about how your body and mind respond to them. This book demonstrates training and qualification for providing direction to those who are not well equipped for solving a problem related to the daily life eating process. This is a short and time-saving opportunity to feel fit and smart yet beautiful internally and externally with the minimum investment ever made.

The following will be used throughout the scripts for ease during the art of narration.

Long pause=10-20 seconds (indicated with L.P and will be given x2 or x3 if used more than once/number of times to be used will be specified)

Middle Pause=5-8 seconds (M.P, other instructions are same as above for frequency)

Short pause=2-3 seconds (S.P, other instructions are same as above for frequency)

1. Meditation for preparation

Let's get ready for a wonderful experience
This experience takes you towards relaxation
The relaxation that you would like to have in your daily routine
You are here, listening to these preparation steps
(S.P after each of the above statements)
You are willing completely to turn your life into success many times more than you already have
You may be doing this for the first time or maybe not
You still tend to feel it a new and rich experience loaded with ease and satisfaction as its outcome
Be favourable to yourself and get started to generously progress into the world, which is full of creative methods to heal
(M.P after each of the above statements)
You are ready now
(L.P)

Whatever you are going through in routine
That is all just a temporary effect of what influence comes to you
You are beyond those worries, hardships, negativity and disappointments
You are taking the hold of converting your losses into profits
The time you have chosen to prepare your body and mind to relax is feasible
You are about to appropriately focus on the existence of yours in this universe

You are going to beautifully touch the possibilities of achieving your dreams
You have the potential to connect with the power of your mind
You can allow creativity to shape your destiny
(M.P after each of the above statements)

Find a comfortable place where you can sit straight or lie down preferably
Make sure your arms and feet are relaxed
It must be easy enough for you to feel the weight of your body on the furniture
You are now grounded with nature
You will transfer the despairs onto the unseen particles of the universe and become light, pure and valuable
Make sure there is no voice around you but you can listen to your heartbeats
Slowly try to close your eyes and dig deep into the world of transformation
(S.PX3 after each of the above statements)
You are going to meditate through all your sensory perceptions
(L.PX2)

Breathing is what you do all the time
Today is the time and opportunity for you to deeply explore and be grateful for what you are capable to do better and notice how it flows
The flow of the breathing making your diaphragm expands and shrinks in a rhythmic manner

You are attentive towards the motion of the natural process with so much power that you rarely recognize before
Today realize how you breathe deeply
Inhale deeply and notice the effect for three seconds, 1, 2, and 3
Hold on and notice the self-control for three seconds, 1, 2, and 3
Exhale and release air for three seconds, 1, 2, and 3
Well done!
(M.PX2 after each of the above statements)

Imagine, there are green grasslands in front of you
You are sitting in the middle of the greens for a long time
You can feel the coldness of the earth and the warmness of the air
The soil is friendly for you and your body temperature is comfortable for exploration of this place
Without any distraction, you are with your eyes closed sitting in a peaceful environment
Notice that your surroundings are safe
You continue to focus on breathing and how the breathing rhythms are mesmerizing your soul
(L.P after each of the above statements)

In the depths of your soul, there is a place like the one you imagine in your surroundings
Get down in the depths of your soul
Imagine there is a staircase leading you to the room of your soul that cooperates with your mind and body *(M.P after each of the above statements)*

With me imagine the movement of your feet from 1-10 on the stairs going down keeping your attention in the middle of your body, 1, 2, 3, 4, 5, 6, 7, 8, 9, 10 (S.P between each)

Now you are at the depth of your soul and the natural green, peaceful place is in front of you

Fresh air is blowing and you continue to breathe deeply

Relaxation is spreading all over your body from the centre of your soul

Your attention is on the centre of your soul where you can feel the relaxation is spreading all over your body

With the progress of each moment, each muscle within your body is getting more and more relaxed

The relaxation is in your muscles spreading from the core of your body to the extremities

(L.P after each of the above statements)

Your stomach is relaxed, your arms are relaxed, and your hands, palms, fingers, nails, chest, neck and face are all relaxed (M.P between each body part)

Relaxation is in your hips, lower back, thighs, legs, feet, heels, soles and toes (M.P between each body part)

Let the thoughts come and go

There is no way to stop them

They are like fresh air and they have no power within themselves

The power is in your attention

Pay attention to your relaxation

You can deep breath and stay relaxed in any situation when the power of your mind focuses on the positivity and happiness, success and achievement, your goals and goals directed action

Mind have thoughts, beliefs and they are rarely factual

Let you free of their influence and deep breathe once again

(M.PX2 after each of the above statements)

Next to your thoughts, you feel emotions

Emotions that are natural, intense and short-lived

You might know your emotions when you react based on them

You are allowed to feel joy, happiness, satisfaction and ease as much as you want

Focus on the moments most of the time in which you laugh openly

Find ways to put a smile on the faces of other people as much as you can

Believe this that you can accept all the love, passion and energy to feel happy

Draw all the positive emotions you have been noticing since childhood

(L.P after each of the above statements)

Let all your actions aligned with your positive emotions

Let all your love direct you to compassion, love and kindness filled acts

Let this introspection of your own experiences flow with the forces that you experience from your surroundings

Notice the enthusiasm and complete familiarity of the internal and external world

The soul and mind works about the body, manifested in actions and behaviours we do all day and night

This appears to establish a connection for better outcomes and productivity

Your productivity determines your success and you are moving ahead to achieve all that you want to achieve

(S.PX2 after each of the above statements)

You must learn the art of managing triggers for moving ahead smoothly

Overcome the challenges by identifying the triggers that stop you from success

The triggers can be managed

They can be a place, a time, an object, a person or an activity that possibly hinders the state of relaxation in your life

You can witness the most relaxed environment daily

Relaxation in the visual scenes in front of your eyes

Relaxation in the voices you hear and the sounds you hear

Relaxation may come with all the textures you touch and the smell you smell and the taste you taste

(S.P after each of the above statements)

Settle yourself to gain control over you completely

Self-control comes with ease as you start to believe that you can control yourself

You may feel the self-control and the power of gaining control all over your mind and body

In all the states of your mental capacity whether it be joy, peace and contentment
Self-control is present there
It progresses and manages to be a part of your actions regularly
You are about to open your existence for a magical and powerful creation of the universe
Let's absorb the deep blessings of health
(M.P after each of the above statements)

Feel the light that is entering every cell of your body to make you comfortable and fully prepared to attain the chain of behaviours that encourages you and stimulates you to progress the relaxation
All the light, a very bright shimmer is now prevailing throughout the body from head to toe and flowing like the thin sheet of water
The light has a soothing effect on your head, the skin of your forehead, feel this light on your cheeks and chin
Feel the light on your neck and shoulders; the light now covers your arms and abdomen
The light now covers your lower body parts
(L.P after each of the above statements)

There is a purpose of the light to spread upon you
It is meant to spread the good virtues, wisdom, patience and morality
It has all that you ever want to seek from the depths of your soul
You are obtaining more and more bravery
You are attaining more and more wisdom
You are more driven to pick the healthy foods

Today is the first day of your journey to pick the food for relaxation
You most of the time eat only for relaxation and you choose to eat only when you are relaxed
(S.P after each of the above statements)

Imagine your real life
The hours in which you feel most pleasure and most fulfilled sense of existence
In real life, you decide to focus on mindfulness all the time
Whatever you do you do it mindfully
You sit, stand, walk, eat, talk, meet and greet people mindfully
You recall the minute details of every hour you spend alive
You do breathing and deep breathing that goes on deeper and deeper for your blood flow to feel
You are indeed at the deepest levels of your peace
Your hair is peace and your perception is peace, your outer is peace and your inner is peace
(S.P after each of the above statements)

Peace is similar to the greenery on which you began imagining the progressive relaxation for your peace
Scan the muscles again for your awareness about how you have built the capacity to relocate peace whenever and wherever you want
You scan your head, face, body and feet; there is a flow of peace and happiness that you have seen
At this point, you are once again witnessing the beauty of nature, the smell of soil, the warm and cold temperatures of the air and grass around you

15

Your body weight has become lighter like a feather and you are ready to fly with the power of your mind
(S.P after each of the above statements)

Coming back to the surface from the depths of your soul is about to happen
When you come back you may apply the peaceful actions as your habit
In all the situations in which you ever live
You can face the challenges with calmness
You are prepared for a bigger achievement and success for the sake of your own life
You potentially get the happiest outcome from this experience as you come along with my voice
Imagine there is a door in the depths of your soul
The place where you are right now
(S.P after each of the above statements)

The same staircase is going upward in the form of 10 stairs (S.P)
You may climb up towards the external world, one at a time, slowly and with peace 1, 2, 3, 4, 5, 6, 7, 8, 9, and 10 (S.P between each number)
Deep breathe as you are out of that staircase in the place of meditation
You have reached the place from where we moved ahead to the glorious success of achieving your ideal body
Open your eyes to the physical objects that are present around you
(M.P after each of the above statements)

You are feeling the heights of your physical and mental competency

With a new perspective to the situations, you daily visit

With a new ambition to meet the people you already know and those who you don't

Your confidence is limitless and there are no boundaries to the exposure

(M.P after each of the above statements)

Praise once your creativity and imagination

Your drive to attract the tolerance and patience

Your self-control is at the peak of your mind

(S.P after each of the above statements)

Your best supply to overcome the barriers to your irrational beliefs is the self-control you have managed to possess (L.P)

Be grateful with open hands, spread arms and say thank you universe!

2. Flexibility in beliefs

Try to sit completely relaxed, as you feel deeply
and deeply relaxed you feel that there is no
distraction around you
The only voice that you hear in your ears is
mine
You need to listen to my voice very carefully
And when you do this, you feel if there are any
voices from your environment, they fade away
Here you must assure yourself that through
following my voice carefully you will not only
benefit from weight loss but also your beliefs
will be flexible while you intend to choose a
food to eat
Get ready for the helpful suggestions and close
your eyes smoothly
(S.P after each of the above statements)

You might imagine your current situation that
you have in your mind about eating healthy and
helpful habits
To dig down deeply into your beliefs imagine
there is are three slopes that are going down
into a basement lounge
Move ahead by choosing one of the slopes that
you can imagine and reach to the lounge that is
extremely comfortable and relaxing
As you pick one of the slopes, move ahead and
by moving forward you may face a large lounge

In this lounge, sit on a sofa with your favourite cloth lining
(L.PX2 after each of the above statements)

Again choose one of your best feelings that you would like to gain through this programming of your mind
To become leaner, smarter, healthier and slimmer
Take a long and deep breath and continue doing it
The best feeling that you choose to focus on today throughout this journey of flexibility in beliefs could be energetic, alert and solid
The feeling that you pick here must be a presenter of your outcome
The outcome that you seek after losing heavy amounts of fat
As you lose more and more fat from your body the weight sheds off
(M.P after each of the above statements)

Pay attention to your deep nice breaths
Let this fat off not only from your body but the mind and your whole life permanently
You can facilitate this process with the help of your beliefs
When you believe you are becoming slimmer because you are losing fat with hypnosis
You would see it coming, now take it easy and comfortable

You are the only person who can make it happen with your willpower and the power of your mind

Into this deep comfortable lounge, you have chosen a feeling that is completely aligned with your belief about yourself following the weight loss

(S.P after each of the above statements)

Imagine a setting where you would like to become flexible

More and more flexible not only physically and psychologically

When your body is flexible you can move freely but when your mind is flexible you can cope with any challenge that comes in your way and interfere with the achievement of goals

Your health goals are as important as your mind

So let your mind be more open, flexible and enjoy the sense of being liberal

Imagine a scene where you would like this change to happen

(S.PX3 after each of the above statements)

Believe it that within the next few minutes, you will recondition your total existence of mind and beliefs

You will turn yourself in a leaner and smarter you

Your eating habits will improve and with your new self-image you will groom your body

Enjoy these moments of change

Imagine your mind is a rubber band and it is
stretching and stretching to a point where it
allows you to insert some very interesting views
that you didn't know
For example, you live not only healthy but
happy as well with your new eating routine
(M.PX2 after each of the above statements)

This place is your mind, all between the stretch
of this rubber band that you imagine you are
allowed to rethink some of the very unhelpful
beliefs that you ever have about your eating
behaviours and can turn them into helpful ones
You will able to enjoy your life in future and
feel satisfied with your eating habits as much as
you were before
Now, pick one of the beliefs that you would like
to change
For this transformation remember to add this
belief into the middle of the stretched rubber
band
(S.P after each of the above statements)

Observe own thoughts, how did they appear in
the first place
Maybe the beliefs come from childhood
experiences
Maybe the beliefs are strengthened by social
pressure
Maybe role models teach the beliefs
Maybe the beliefs are the results of
experimentation in your teenage

There may be hundreds of reasons and possible combination and interaction of factors behind it
You are still free to flexible your beliefs
Focus on imagining an alternative to the belief you have picked to transform today
In the middle of the rubber band, your belief becomes flexible
(S.P after each of the above statements)

Identify the various effects of the irrational belief that you have chosen to insert into a rubber band
It might have changed the way you look at your body
It might have influenced your eating habits
It might have modified your view about your life
Now imagine stretching that rubber band a bit more
As you stretch the rubber band you feel that the band is getting more and more glossy and beautiful
As the band gets more beautiful you feel that your belief towards unhelpful eating is reforming into a helpful one
(S.P after each of the above statements)

Challenge the unhelpful belief at this point now focus again
As you stretch the rubber band you feel that the band is getting more and more glossy and beautiful

As the band gets more beautiful you feel that
your belief towards unhelpful eating is
reforming into a helpful
If you have believed that eating more than
needed to keep you away from food for longer
hours
Challenge this unhelpful and irrational belief
with this affirmation
Eating only when hungry and only healthy
keeps my stomach filled and satisfied for 4-6
hours
(S.P after each of the above statements)

Finding alternatives is an amazing way to create
flexible beliefs
There is always more than one way to think
about a situation
The need for food is physiological
There is no relation of food requirement with
the time to eat
It varies for everyone in different situations
There is a much more helpful way to eat as
intended by nature
Eating the amount of food equals to our fist and
so on
The extra storage of fat is the result of eating
more than required by the body
So, here one of the beliefs is flexible for your
help in transforming the body from fat-
containing to healthy
(S.P after each of the above statements)

Now you have experienced how to think in dialects

Thinking in a dialectical manner means thinking in two different dimensions for your ease

You might consider a belief negatively and then needs to rethink to make it positive

Whenever you feel the need to imagine an alternative and flexible belief

Imagine a rubber band stretched to an extent that you could put it in an old belief to generate options

In this way, your flexibility in beliefs grow even more and more

(S.P after each of the above statements)

Affirm your capacity to lose weight and fat by eating less and less than you burn

Eat fewer calories than you burn

Eat less fat than you loose

Day by day try to follow this rule

Eating into the limits of body requirements would also enable you to think in different dialects

Adjusting the meal according to fewer calories and measuring food for less fat and more proteins or less simple carbohydrates and more complex carbohydrates excite your mind for more alternatives to prepare and consume the food

(S.P after each of the above statements)

Becoming open-mindedness is like a rubber band stretched at ease without any force or difficulty
Your mind is also a rubber band and it works like one at least to reprogram into a new you
A new you are a healthy eater, a healthy cook and a healthy person with complete satisfaction
To reduce weight, gather some flexible beliefs about how to meet your body requirements without much food
And repeat this pattern until you achieve your ideal weight and figure
The inert fat needs to be released and the daily food must not exceed what you released
As you take part in this initiative you will feel much more potential in you
(S.P after each of the above statements)

Focus again on your own beliefs about food and weight and your body image
Learn to be mindful of your beliefs daily few minutes
Spend few minutes before you try to eat something
What do you think of the food you eat?
Observe all the experiences that elicit your mind related to your eating habits
It can be related to the quantity of food or quality of food or the outcome of the food you intend you eat
(S.P after each of the above statements)

Settle your thoughts that come to your mind into the rubber band and rethink to reprogram the thoughts
This is one of the easiest ways to seek flexibility in your beliefs and allowing yourself to think in different aspects
As an outcome, you observe each day that how you make a difference in your eating habits and overall self-image
As compared to your past your some of the beliefs have now rescreened for a better future
You are a quick learner and I have complete trust in your competency to achieve an ideal weight
(S.P after each of the above statements)

Remember, no matter what procedure would you use for measuring the food you eat in terms of calories and fat
A weight scale is also a flexible tool
Note that you are going to continue a flexible journey
The measurement varies for everyone and depending on your activity and circumstances plus the food quality
Find a variety of options for your measured diet and support a good storage system for the leftovers
Whatever you do the only thing you need to focus on is flexibility both mentally and physically

So now do more brainstorming, create new cells, move your body freely and survive at your best
(S.P after each of the above statements)

Coming back from the world of flexibility
Be grateful for few seconds towards your capacity to reach here
You have decided to allow more flexibility in your beliefs and storing more food in the fridge than in your body
At your convenience, you are doing good at a great deal
Cut off the past and start a new day for a better tomorrow with the patterns of healthy eating
(S.P after each of the above statements)

As you have understood the easy and quick method to seek flexibility in beliefs
Again take a sweet and slow breath
Feel rested and deeply rested as much as you can
You are getting lighter and lighter like air in the balloon with readiness to turn your beliefs about food from irrational to rational
You seem prepared to get action on your food eating patterns
(S.P after each of the above statements)

You might imagine the same lounge you started in
In this lounge, you are on a sofa with your favourite cloth lining

Take a look at the lounge and find the slopes to go back upwards from the depths and dungeons of your mind where all your beliefs are deeply rooted

Imagine there is are three slopes that are going upward back into your place where you began listening to my voice

Move ahead by choosing one of the slopes that you can imagine and reach safely

As you pick one of the slopes, move ahead and by moving forward you may feel relieved and lighter

Open your eyes and you are ready to take action on your healthy life

(L.PX2 after each of the above statements)

3. Placing the gastric band

Settle yourself to a place where you feel most comfortable
This is the continuation of a wonderful journey towards success
This is your success and you can attain the completion of your desires
The desires that you have been asking for fulfilment is now very close to your presence
You are about to achieve a desirable body weight to your satisfaction
You are going to satisfy yourself with the best ideal body image that you always wanted to have
You are mentally prepared to receive the gift of the universe that you have been yearning for a lot for months
(M.P after each of the above statements)

Make sure you are present on soft bedding or sofa in a room full of quietness
Let the position of your body completely loose and stay straight to feel all the weight of your body completely resting on the furniture
As you feel relaxed and your body gets heavy, your eyes are becoming heavy
Continue feeling the heaviness on your eyelids
Now close your eyes softly and tighten the closed eyes
The eyes are getting tighter and tighter as you close them

You are going to experience a warm change in your beautiful body
(S.P after each of the above statements)

Imagine you are on the first step of your success ladder
This step is warm and welcoming for you
To change what you want to change in your body feel the warmness to the depths of your core
The middle of your body is the powerhouse for transformation
Get more and more relaxed as you breathe rhythmically (Repeat twice)
(S.P after each of the above statements)

Let you breathe deeper and deeper as you imagine the sea breeze coming towards your face and touch your skin politely
There is a peace that flows everywhere in a pattern spreading all over your body in a form of a network

Notice that pattern for relaxation
That is providing relaxation in your head, ears, face, eyes, neck, shoulders, arms, hands, palms, fingers, chest, stomach, thighs, lower back, legs, feet, toes and heels (S.P after each body part)
You are feeling relaxed in each of your body parts and muscles are getting looser and looser that allows you to feel completely free for a change
Your body might lay straight with an erect spine
As you observe the natural curve of your backbone at the back of your body weight

You notice how the relaxation is flowing in a rhythmic pattern all over your body as naturally as possible
(L.P after each of the above statements)

Try to inhale as much deeper as possible
Through your nose, you inhale for three seconds
Then you hold the breathing for three seconds
Then you exhale for three seconds and blow the air out gradually and completely
Continue this process and you may feel how the lungs get full with fresh air as you inhale and the stomach spreads out as well
Upon exhale, your stomach shrinks and lungs flatten as the air goes out of your mouth in a flow
Through this process, the body parts feel the relief from tension to relaxation, from tightness to calmness and looseness
(S.P after each of the above statements)

Bundles of oxygen arrive in each cell of your body with inhaling
And the carbon dioxide, impure air and toxins leave out from your body through exhaling
You are completely aware of the feeling when the stomach shrinks and moves towards the back of your body near the backbone
The flesh of your stomach appears flat and as you imagine it gets flat and flat as much as you need
You are full of energy and positivity with the hope and ease of feeling a flat stomach throughout your life
(M.P after each of the above statements)

31

Today is the day to realize the ideal image is very close to you and as you desire more about it imagine more about it

It will get closer and you feel that your stomach flatness is in your control

As you want to feel your stomach the extra fat is shedding off your stomach area

You have taken the responsibility to burn the fat off your body from all over the body parts that are loaded with the excessive body fat

Affirm this change for your body that you love the most "I am bringing the change in my body for a flat physique and fat burning attitude" (Repeat)

(L.P after each of the above statements)

Remind yourself that "I do for my body what I want and I feel love and kindness towards my body, I accept my body as it is flattening and reaching to the desired shape and desired weight".

Affirm as you are in the deepest relaxation

Imagine yourself in a state around a soothing breeze

You are in a camp with mountains full of green grass all over the way you look

The camp has deep light and flame contains a scent of rose

The tent of the camp is a shimmer as if stars are all above your skin

(S.P after each of the above statements)

Absorbing this mesmerizing scent, the mountains are sprinkling snow

The snow seems to glow like a purple tint of the sky
The tip of the sky looks glorious and secure
In this wonderful cosy mood of the surroundings
You spread your arms to invite the ideal image of yours
Keep looking at this site and clench your fist once very tight
As quickly as possible now release the tightness and let your fears go away
All of your muscles are relaxed and loose
The body is deeply loose and heavy at the centre of the stomach
(L.P after each of the above statements)

As you try to go down deeper in your body walk down towards the centre in ten steps with my voice
1
2
3
4
5
5
6
7
8
9
10
You are on the deepest end of the centre of your body
Move few steps and take a complete view of your destination

This is where you want a change, a transformation and this is where you need to relax
As you are willing to change your body delightfully
Seek the help of this universe and let the power functions for your desire fulfilment
Let the senses perceive the stomach at the deepest level
(S.P after each of the above statements)

You agree with your body to freely let go of the emotional and physical burden harmlessly
The load you have been carrying is swishing away as you embrace a gastric band around your stomach with an open heart
Accept the gastric band on this place of your stomach where most of the weight, burden and fat lives
A gastric band is placed along your waistline
This is the same part where your physical, mental and emotional exhaustion are placed as well that you have been experiencing so far
This gastric band influences your fat burning, accelerates the vanishing of undesirable pounds and reduce your tendency to gain undesirable weight on your stomach
(M.P after each of the above statements)

Be aware of your body there is a gastric band on your stomach
You have accepted that gastric band and you adjust to it

You are mindful and ready to maximize the
happiness that this gastric band placement is
offering you
Imagine the gastric band on your stomach visually;
listen to your breathing with a gastric band placed
on your stomach
Feel the gastric band is glowing and soft
You are in love with this tiny band around your
stomach
(M.PX2 after each of the above statements)

And as you meet the gastric band closely you may
feel the optimal sense of health, courage and energy
As you observe the gastric band, your curiosity
extends
A vivid sketch of the gastric band is a thin and
small belt
Let me discuss with you that the gastric band is
placed around your stomach in your favourite
colour
This band is perfect somewhat larger than the size
of your fist
The gastric band's colour gives you joy and the
texture of the gastric band is flashing as if you are
seeing an entertaining screen
The gastric band is of your choice
You choose the gastric band that is best for you
(S.P after each of the above statements)

The placement of the gastric band is a success for
you
Your first success in the best shape that you love

Notice the gastric band is placed exactly on the position where it is needed to restrict the amount of food you eat daily
Your daily food consumption is getting smaller and smaller in portion but more and more delicious and nutritious
As the process of eating slows down for you
You recognize the fullness, lightness and usefulness of the food that you eat throughout the day only when you are hungry
(S.PX2 after each of the above statements)

The gastric band placed around your stomach on the area where fat is in excess
The gastric band is making your stomach smaller and flatter
This gastric band is the solution to treat your body weight without any medical procedure
The gastric band is creative that motivates you to manage your weight effortlessly
All around your stomach your gastric band is helping in the quick digestion of your food
You get the nutrients from your daily food
Concentrate on the skin of your stomach
The skin is getting tighter and tighter to support the internal organs as the fat burns out and release from the stomach area
(S.PX3 after each of the above statements)

Imagine the fat-releasing out of all other areas of your body
As you feel fat burns the body feels lighter and there is little hunger that you feel afterwards

Each time you eat, you eat only a small portion of healthy and natural food
The sources of food that you buy usually is free of fats, sodium and simple sugar
Anytime you can eat your favourite food
Continue focusing on the gastric band placed on your stomach
Whenever you feel hungry and eat something you enjoy with the presence of the gastric band
Identify the signs of hunger in your body that signals you to eat
(S.PX4 after each of the above statements)

There are signs that signals to stop eating when you eat
Listen to the full stomach feeling
The gastric band minimizes your eating because now you eat only the adequate amount of food that your body needs
You are ready to live a healthy life
This gives you a feeling of satisfaction, fulfilment and happiness
Your mind is relaxed, your body is calm and your stomach flattens as you closely observe the gastric band placement for your good
Once again appreciate the benefits of the gastric band that is placed on your stomach
(S.P after each of the above statements)

Take a deep breath and recall the presence of your concentration on the core of your stomach area with the most body fat

This accumulation is now getting out from the
depths of your stomach
This amazes you as if you are on a vacation
There is a camp in which you are resting
Noticing the sky and allowing the tiny snowdrops
letting you feel cold and calm
The gastric band supply you with deeper
observation skills, awareness and mindful
appreciation of the slightest changes under the skin
of your stomach
Your total body weight lessens and gives you
admiration for choosing it as your lifestyle
(S.P after each of the above statements)

Wherever you go this gastric band stays with you
You can sit, stand, sleep, eat and do all the routine
tasks with this gastric band
This band is like a piece of cloth on your skin
As you move it stays with you
You are comfortable with this gastric band
It gives you an ideal body image and your desirable
feelings of beauty
The gastric band is a part of your body
You are thankful for this choice of yours
You make decisions for yourself and the decisions
are good for your health
(S.P after each of the above statements)

Come back from the depths of your core
Your body is reached to a state of fitness without
any undesirable effect
Come up to the surroundings where you
comfortably lay down on a smooth surface

As you hear my voice counting 10-1 imagine
yourself getting out of the deepness of your
stomach at the core of your body
10
9
8
7
6
5
4
3
2
1
Here you are in your new world where you can see
the most soothing objects of nature
There is a natural smell of the air around you
You can feel the taste of your pleasure
Listen to any sound that you can hear
Move ahead to a fresh start.
(S.P after each of the above statements)

4. Affirmations for self-satisfaction

Let's get relaxed
It is a blessing to sit relaxed
Every day we strive to get better and better
Just like that strive to get more and more deeply
relaxed
This is the time to leave your hands and palms
completely open and allow yourself to receive the
most useful and blessed sense of self-satisfaction
within you
Self-satisfaction is grown daily and makes you the
best version of yourself
As you know that in this world we all try to become
the best version of ourselves to achieve the best
With full of adventurous experiences and incredible
knowledge you can grab the satisfaction you seek
(S.P after each of the above statements)

In whatever position you are
Become the most relaxed person on earth
Loosen your limbs
Loosen your body
Make sure you are wearing loose and soft clothes
Your bedding is soft and you are breathing in and
out with the deepest inhale and exhale movements
Nice
Focus on relaxation once again and scan all your
body parts one by one from head to toe if there are
any tensions simply contract those muscles and
count for three seconds

Now release and smile nicely, openly and deeply
(S.P after each of the above statements)

Pay attention to your eyes
Make sure the light is dim in your room
Make sure there is no distraction around you
Your eyes are getting heavier and heavier as you
continue breathing
Breathing with heavy eyes is making your eyes
even heavier
Don't try to blink your eyes
Avoid blinking and let it imagine that you are
sleeping to deeply feel the feelings of satisfaction
As few movements pass you feel that the eyes are
about to close
Now as it feels difficult to keep the eyes open
Close them tightly and make you relaxed
(S.P after each of the above statements)

Imagine the eating patterns that you usually observe
in yourself
These patterns might mostly let you eat more than
your body needs
Excessive eating makes your food store extra
calories more easily
The carbohydrates when in excess they are also
stored in your body in the form of fats
Similarly, the fat is stored in the form of fats and
your body becomes bigger and bigger than the ideal
one
To combat this outcome we seek satisfaction
We need to readily feel satisfied with the amount of
the food we eat

41

(S.P after each of the above statements)

You may have an idea that the amount of food you
used to eat in the past didn't satisfy you earlier
Even there might be some times when the food you
consumed didn't satisfy you at all
Lack of knowledge about food consumption may
become a barrier between you and your weight loss
But you are now ready to turn your dissatisfaction
into satisfaction
Whatever you do and feel and eat is totally in your
hands
Your wisdom tells you that you can feel totally
satisfied when you begin eating healthy and
emerged yourself as a completely new person
(S.P after each of the above statements)

Imagine now to satisfy yourself, your hunger, your
stomach and your body needs with the help of
eating less and burning more calories and fats
You continue losing fat and excessive calories by
eating lesser and lesser
This becomes a regular compulsion for you to eat
lesser and burn more fat calories
In this way, your fat stores are ended and you will
come out as a slimmer, leaner and healthier you
Replace the old patterns of eating more and burning
fewer calories and fat off your skin with eating less
and burning more and more calories and fats
Imagine your extra weight pounds are now melting
and melting and melting with great intensity

With the eyes of your mind, you are capable to see
yourself satisfied deeply with the image of yourself
that is now relaxed, calm, healthy and slim
There is plenty of food but you feel satisfied
There are plenty of choices but you intend to pick
only those with the lowest calories possible
You enjoy drinking water at ease
You love colourful fruits and vegetables in small
portions
Because you are satisfied with them deeply
(S.P after each of the above statements)

Planning and setting goals for your healthy life in
advance is one of the most beneficial tricks to keep
your mouth open for healthy foods only and only at
the time of need
Chew the freshest and raw foods with lots of
vitamins and minerals and that is all you need most
of the time
Then along with it, you have a choice to pick
lightly cooked, boiled or grilled lean meat and
olives to accompany the whole-wheat bun
Add some greens, seeds and nuts to make it even
more exotic and you are satisfied with one of your
daily meals
(S.P after each of the above statements)

Taking actions upon your goals is not to shame but
to feel pride
This proud you do in your decision making is the
satisfaction
There is satisfaction in every sip of your water if
you explore

There is satisfaction in each bite of the food you must consume if you wish to observe
Making a daily habit to write the food observations and eating experiences in a journal by the end of the day is an excellent to practice self-satisfaction
(S.P after each of the above statements)

Evaluating alternatives is another step to achieve satisfaction with your food
This is an honour to take part in your food practices
Leave the worries and avail the accessible choices to pick and pack for your bag
Participate in the storage of your healthy food in the forms of bites; fingers and crisps within zip-lock plastic bags
These tiny bags are good to invest within for your most valuable life
Even if you put the smallest bite in your bag from your leftover veggies and corn burrito or a cutlet you will be able to burn little calories and at least avoiding the addition of many more calories that are not required between the meals and before the eating timings by not buying anything unhealthy from the market when you are away from home and your regular food storage
With tiny portions of healthy food, you would be able to manage your odd cravings and appetite
When these cravings and appetite are satisfied your body stays safe permanently from the damage you intend you make with a packaged food
Few choices can save you from impulsive acts of binge eating and addictive artificial flavours
(S.P after each of the above statements)

Affirmations to bring a positive shift in body and mind must always be filled in your routine
Read them, write them, recall them, memorize them, remind them or verbalize them, paste them around you in written form with a suitable motivating image or draw yourself, keep them in your file, pocket or drawer they have the sensitive power to self-hypnotize you and satisfy at the deepest level
Some of them are "I have willingness and determination to manage my cravings and controlling my binge eating episodes, sizes are only numbers they don't define me, I believe that matters"
(S.P after each of the above statements)

Keep moving and repeat it with me with more focus and attention, slowly and with understanding
Register each of these words one by one
"I have willingness and determination to manage my cravings and controlling my binge eating episodes, sizes are only numbers they don't define me, I believe that matters"
Register each of these words one by one
"I have willingness and determination to manage my cravings and controlling my binge eating episodes, sizes are only numbers they don't define me, I believe that matters" (Now repeat each word with S.P)
You do it great now for the one last time say
"I have willingness and determination to manage my cravings and controlling my binge eating

episodes, sizes are only numbers they don't define me, I believe that matters"
This was one of the astonishing dares that you just passed brilliantly and beautifully
The courage and the bravery that you have is mostly the care you show to yourself
As you feel more and more satisfied with your body and self-image the self-satisfaction flows in and out of your heart enlightening you and those around you glamorously
(S.P after each of the above statements)

Achievement of dreams is possible if you care about your peace go for your dreams
Visualize your dream of achieving satisfaction daily
Observe and describe the characteristics of your ideal satisfaction
Note the related emotions, beliefs, words, symbols and let yourself love the art of giving and receiving with this exchange of dreams with reality
This idea is fantastic and so does you
(S.P after each of the above statements)

Success in satisfaction is any act of kindness that you show towards yourself and others
It can be selecting a clever food or tantalizing natural herb for your meal
It can be a lovely, outstanding and wonderful dish that you cook for a friend
Or it can be an extra bag of chips or any other unhealthy food that you donate to someone in need

All of this shows you satisfaction to give something
and in return, you may receive bundles of
satisfaction
Forget the past mistakes they matter no more
There is nothing more beautiful than the path of
success to achieve a thread to hold and follow your
dreams
(S.P after each of the above statements)

With the solid belief in your food-making skills and
ability to use natural food for health creatively
Make a pout to fly a soft kiss away from your
mouth in the universe as a token of thanks for
guiding you to success and satisfaction
Be restful and peaceful to every bit of your body,
each inch of your skin and the minute cells, your
organs and the blood flowing within
(S.P after each of the above statements)

Settle your mind to take in the above-given
suggestions deeply to root in your mind
Your mind sees the images of the optimal
satisfaction that you seek in your daily life for your
body and eating habits
Whatever you do you feel satisfied and succeeded,
there is plenty of hope and positivity in your beliefs
as you affirm the self-satisfaction and understand
the mechanism of feeling satisfied the level of your
satisfaction exceeds moment by moment without
any hurdles
It doesn't matter how you temporarily feel but the
satisfaction matters with the long-term effect and
influence on your mind and soul

(S.P after each of the above statements)

Now again focus on the relaxation that has reached
the depths of your body
Feel that you are the most relaxed person on earth
Your limbs are loose and your body is loose,
weightless and carefree
You breathe in and out with the deepest inhale and
exhale movements
Nice
Focus on relaxation one last time and scan all your
body parts one by one from head to toe if there are
any tensions simply contract those muscles and
count for three seconds
Now release and smile nicely, openly and deeply
(S.P after each of the above statements)

You may open your eyes now and manifest the
visualization with your perception
As you are satisfied you feel much more love and
tenderness for your body and you treat it with a
recovered self-satisfaction, the past leaves off the
corner of your mind
You are worthy enough to put effort and time into
the planning of food that you eat
You attend to your body weight and shape and you
stop running from it but you own it as it is and feel
its beauty with the most compassionate eyes that
have unconditional love and empty judgments
(S.P after each of the above statements)

5. Embrace your emotions

Find an area in your home with dim lights
Choose a place with the least noises around you
Choose a place without any visual distractions
Get yourself ready for a pleasurable experience
containing a lot of sensory outcomes
Become relaxed in a situation where you get easily
engaged in the process of visualizing and
manifesting your ideal emotional stability
Take a look at some point in front of you
Maybe a wall where you can focus for a long time
Try to open your eyes without blinking as much as
you can
Let your eyes close gently when you feel they are
tired
Take your time
(L.PX2 after each of the above statements)

As you feel your eyes are closed and you can
experience the feelings that are associated with
your current emotional status
Whatever your feelings are let them go
Release the clutter of your mind that have been
upsetting you for a long time
Try to feel most comfortable and recall an event
from your life that previously and effortlessly
caused you laughter
Remember that laughter
Imagine your voices of laughing and your facial
expressions

Notice the textures you felt that time and the movements of your overall posture
(L.PX2 after each of the above statements)

Suppose that your desire to become slim and slender is a realistic wish
Still, look at your emotions that are associated with this desire
I count till seven and you would notice some of the emotions that elicited by the idea of this desire
1
2
3
4
5
6
7
To be honest, most of the emotions and feelings attached to this desire may be negative
As they can be shame, guilt, disappointment and hopelessness
This is natural due to the failures in the past to achieve this desire
(L.P after each of the above statements)

Take a nice deep breath for three seconds
1
2
3
And realize, on the other hand, the emotions associated with the desire to become slim and slender might be positive for example, hope, success, happiness, satisfaction

Now try to feel more and more deeply and deeply calm

This is just the start of your recognition for this emotional stability possibility that you might have resisted so far

Achieving emotional stability and peace is a skill to learn, master and practice

Continue focusing on your breathing once again
(S.P after each of the above statements)

Your emotions are the triggers for your actions
Emotions are also very intense but short-lived
But the impact they would have on your mental health is long-term

Feel the intensity of the emotions that you feel when you look at the food

Feel the intensity of the emotions that you feel when you avoid certain foods

Feel the intensity of the emotions that you feel when you look at your body weight

Feel the intensity of the emotions that you feel when you feel something about your physique
(S.P after each of the above statements)

Depth of all the emotions that you have just tried to look at is the real feelings that may be good or bad

All kinds of such feelings are very much strong and the potential of these emotions can make your stability stick to your healthy diet or can break your integrity with your outlook towards food

The emotions that you have just identified can be a motivator or a breaker of your healthy food routine

Yes, this is for your awareness to manage your emotions wisely for the best weight loss outcomes
(S.P after each of the above statements)

What you think of yourself also elicits an emotion
Imagine the feeling when you look at yourself in the mirror
Imagine the feeling when you look at your food plate on the dining table
Imagine the feeling when you look at your wardrobe and pick a dress to wear
Imagine the feeling when you look at yourself in a picture from a party
All these emotions that are related to different events are actually what lead you to a healthy routine following or unhealthy routine following
(S.P after each of the above statements)

Are there myths that are attached to your emotions and food?
Now observe and get ready to identify and challenge those myths
For example dissatisfaction with the weight reduction
Weight reduction is a moment to cherish and celebrate with the motivation to keep following a healthy routine
Challenge this myth with the following affirmation and correct the falsely held belief
"I am satisfied with my body and weight as it is, I love myself and my healthy routine because it is fruitful for my overall health in the long-term"
Now take a deep nice breath

(S.P after each of the above statements)

You are separate from negative emotions
When you are satisfied with your eating healthy foods behaviour then there is no point in feeling low and disappointed because of it
You need to sort out such contradictions
This is okay to face a contradiction due to separate beliefs and actions but emotions are the glue that connects them very well
Feel that you are becoming more and more slender
It shows that you are happy about it
You are satisfied with the eating behaviours and new foods that you freshly add to your grocery
(S.P after each of the above statements)

Loving-kindness in your heart is a tool to align your emotions and actions in a row following by flexible and positive beliefs
As you chose to eat healthy foods remember that you love your body and you are kind towards your health by doing this
You eat protein for strength and take up most of the water with minerals and vitamins packed food in smaller quantities possible to fit your stomach needs
All of this process is the part of your positive emotions towards yourself
The positive emotions guide you to fill your plate with smaller portions of food
(S.P after each of the above statements)

Colours that spread from your love and kindness towards your body has spread all around your meal Imagine the colours that you see in lean meats, the rainbow colours that you see in the vegetables, the fruits, the nuts and seeds, the colours that you see in food before peeling and after you peel
You would like to pick some of the foods in your hands and you enjoy how they touch your skin and settle against the softness of your fingers and palms
Open yourself to all the colours in your healthy foods list to set away from the preferences
(S.P after each of the above statements)

Facilitate others in compassion
Play a shared game
Share your food with your loved ones, family members even classmates and anyone who you meet daily
Spread the loving and kindness of your emotional energies outside your body influences
Spreading love and sharing kindness with others often gives you an abundance
The abundance of food, the abundance of health, the abundance of gratitude and the abundance of getting more and more attractive with the emotional stability and self-control
Spread all the good around you and then become ready to get it back in larger quantity from the universe
(S.P after each of the above statements)

Observe that loving and kindness towards yourself and others is making you stronger emotionally

This practice for your emotions benefits you in managing the emotional eating at times

This practice for your emotions stops you from the emotional eating out of boredom or relationship conflicts

This practice for your emotions benefits you in managing the eating unhealthy food or any food in excess

The harmful eating is most of the times the emotional eating

Negative emotions in the background water the actions that hazard your healthy eating practice
(S.P after each of the above statements)

You choose food with a wise mind

You prefer to attain a balance in your diet

The balance in your diet and selection of daily healthy foods is a part of the rational process

The rational process is done by our wise mind that is separated from the emotional mind

When our emotions are managed we can think with a wise mind

Your body tends to choose the foods that give strength and build muscle mass rather than the storage of fats in abundance

Our body craves for fat no more and there will be no additional fat intake and rarely the fat is stored
(S.P after each of the above statements)

You do mindful eating whenever you can identify your emotional triggers and calm them down before choosing foods to eat

Affirm, "I feel strong and free of any heavy fats and starches or sugary foods"
As you affirm feel that there is no appetite for unhealthy foods in your stomach
Imagine and say to yourself that I feel no need to eat sweets
I dislike fat and creams
I have no desire for butter
I don't like ice creams and candies
(S.P after each of the above statements)

Observe and affirm that I eat no excessive food
I eat only when hungry
I take small food bites
I taste and smell the food very well
I see the food and listen to the chew of my food and the bites I take
I eat only a small amount of food
The foods that are unhealthy elicit unpleasant emotions in me and I eat only those foods that give me pleasure
I take my time to enjoy the flavours of the food I consider healthy
I am satisfied with my positive emotions and I focus on skimmed milk and low-fat cheese with low caloric foods
(S.P after each of the above statements)

Continue affirming to yourself that my emotions are not interfering with my food intake
I eat only healthy foods regardless of my emotional experiences

I manage my emotions and allow myself to feel the taste of all the healthy foods completely

I feel much better when I eat in small bites

A small number of foods provide me more value to my goals about a healthy and fit lifestyle

I weigh myself because I am hoping that fat has been shed and weight has been decreased

I want to look attractive and I am making myself attractive more and more as I continue eating better than before

(S.P after each of the above statements)

I only respond to the needs of my body

I am managing my emotions for feeling better and to eat better

Whenever I weigh there is a decrease of a couple of pounds

This happens because I follow a healthy eating and I keep it separate from my emotions

My emotional energies cannot be compensated with my eating habits

I learn to eat easily without the influence of my emotions

I stay mindful always when I eat

(S.P after each of the above statements)

What I get from being a mindful eater is that I can enjoy my life even more with healthy eating

Healthy eating is making my sleep better, my digestion is improved and my overall quality of life is improved

I have improved my skin glow and texture; my skin feels fresh and clear

I feel less clutter in my mind and I manage my stress

I maintain my confidence that boost my motivation

I am doing daily pleasurable activities to keep my energy levels up with less consumption of food and more water intake

I am greatly thankful for this process

(S.P after each of the above statements)

Open your eyes quickly and look at the same point you focused on in the beginning to restore the power of positive emotions you have experienced so far

Tomorrow just

Enjoy a single slice of dark and coarse bread in breakfast

Balance your nutrients by eating a green vegetable in lunch

Blend the dinner with yellow corns and red beans

Mix and experiment with the exotic tasty foods that are available to serve for your health and gathered directly from nature as they mature

(S.P after each of the above statements)

6. Tightening the gastric band

Prepare yourself to get comfortable for a beautiful venture
This venture covers the time in which you can make a lot of change in yourself
Your wish is about to fulfil and a goal is near to achieve
You gracefully and with ease learn the art of staying relaxed and beneficial for your good
Ideal body weight in your mind is manifesting in your real life
You are getting a slim waist and a leaner body, a flat stomach that is coming in your path with satisfying outcomes
Moving forward your satisfaction is the most valuable outcome that is taken into consideration
Slowly, very slowly, you can allow yourself at this moment to peacefully rest against a piece of furniture where you relax deeply
(S.P after each of the above statements)

As you hear my voice, simply straight the back of the body and transfer the weight on the chair or bed wherever you get involved in the transformation without any distraction
Close your eyes as soon as you find yourself calm
As you get your eyes closed tightly feel the heaviness of your body and eyes
Continue paying attention to the surroundings in which you are resting

There is no voice around you, your inner self and outer self there is only calmness
A deep calming sensory perception of yourself at the moment is all in your focus
(S.P after each of the above statements)

Let your mind empty
Vacant your mind from unnecessary ideas
Focus on your sensations of the body
The sensations are all over your body
Let the ideas float off your mind and pay attention to your muscles
Your muscles are absorbing deep relaxation in your head, your ears, your face, your eyes, your neck, shoulders, arms, hands, palms and fingers, your abdomen and your back, your legs and feet and toes and the heels, they are all getting more and more relaxed
As you are deeply relaxed, you are completely focused on the breathing pattern of your lungs
(L.P after each of the above statements)

As you release air from your mouth your body shrinks
As you inhale once again your nose fetches air into the lungs and the chest expands
As I count from one to three, continue paying attention to your breathing pattern
Once, two and three
You feel that breathing is getting deeper and deeper to allow deeper relaxation all around your body
You are motivated enough to stay relaxed and you observe the chest and belly movements

Place one hand of yours on your chest, other on
your belly that has the gastric band
(M.P after each of the above statements)

Now confidently breathe as deep as you can and
feel it for few seconds
Your hopes are high and your energy is positive
With this power in your mind imagine yourself
going down deeper into the depths of your body
At the core where your gastric band is placed
Where the desirable changes are taking place
I repeat the numbers from one to ten and you feel
yourself moving deeper into the cells of your body
as a direct observer
One
Two
Three
Four
Five
Six
Seven
Eight
Nine
Ten
This is the same place where your gastric band is
tied like a belt around your stomach
(S.P after each of the above statements)

At this depth of your core, the vibes are passionate
This shows your willingness to become a successful
achiever

Your acceptance is powerful and your attitude towards the gastric band slimness is quite affirmative

One more time affirms, "The change in my body weight is in my control"

Yes believe this that you are attracting the desired body weight, desired body shape and you are getting rid of the unnecessary fat with your muscles

The fat that weighs you down

The fat that has started leaving your body since you put the magical gastric band on your body with excessive belly fat

(M.P after each of the above statements)

This point on your body where the gastric band is placed

You open yourself to bring change

There is no magic but it works like magic

The burden has been released from your belly

Your belly is converted into a slimmer place where the muscles are getting toned

This is happening in the manner you want

Your desire to have smooth change is now getting on a deeper level

Stay true to your commitment to change and continue focusing on the change you desire

The gastric band become tighter than before in the next few minutes

Keep noticing the slightest changes that your body makes

It can be a feeling of lightness after you consume food

You may smell the relaxing scents from the air you breathe
The air around you touches your skin like a weightless feather
The taste of your healthy food choices feels good
Even the sight of your food appears appealing regardless of the choice of food is natural and raw
These sensations are soothing as you feel that clean air is helping with your breathing in symphony like rhythms
There is indeed a whole scenario builds to favour your comfort with the gastric band
(L.P after each of the above statements)

Welcome to the next level of your inner self
Note the voice of your core
The core pleasantly directs you to comes out of your mind and experience the body at its deepest end
At this resting state, shining light is evident for you to imagine the gastric band tied around your stomach
It sticks to your skin and spread like a belt covering all that is undesirable in your life
Your body image is improved, as you stay aware of the gastric band protection from the unpleasant experiences
You might have heard the criticism that is no more a part of your life with the help of the gastric band your positive emotions are maximized
(S.P after each of the above statements)

This is wonderful that your body is secure and the gastric band has been changing your attitude towards the responses from the outer world
You are in charge of your feelings, you choose only and you choose only the pleasurable ones
Imagine the cheerfulness of your smile as the placement of gastric band has dropped half of the weight that you ever want to get rid of yourself
You are still losing a couple of inches off your body
(S.P after each of the above statements)

Take that shining light with your observation towards all the cells of your stomach
This stomach has lesser weight today than before
There are lesser layers of fat cells
There is a strong glittery shine that gives you hope and confidence
Let your cells relaxed a little bit more and breathe deeper as you imagine every inch of your skin
Your skin all around your body previously containing fat is healing
The healing is spreading from the centre of your body
At the centre, you have the gastric band and with that gastric band on your waistline you have power
(M.P after each of the above statements)

The gastric band's power is shining even brighter
The light is getting brighter and brighter that it fully covers your core and cells within your body
Feel the tightness of the gastric band, as the light gets brighter

The bright light calms down your senses and muscles with tightening of the gastric band around your tummy

The slightest tightening of the gastric band is gradually becoming thick

As you feel the small size gastric band is slowly pressing the skin of your stomach even closer to the back of your body

This gastric band is your favourite

The colour of the gastric band is your most desirable one

(S.P after each of the above statements)

Continue the picture of the gastric band in your imagination

The tightness of the gastric band is at an acceptable level

Allow yourself to relax

Your body is completely loose and the gastric band tightness is still allowing you to move flawlessly

This is another positive achievement of your appearance that the gastric band is tightened on your stomach and you are feeling happy

Take few steps ahead and embrace this change freely

With the flat stomach, the tightness of the gastric band is suitable for you to physically rest, turn and move, sit and walk

(L.PX2 after each of the above statements)

Your choice to accept a tighter gastric band is one of the best decisions for your health

The gastric band tightness increases your motivation to lose weight and burns even more fat residues

The tighter gastric band saves you from other methods

Your time is saved as you get to benefit from your tighter gastric band quickly and effortlessly

The gastric band is less complicated and full of ease

As you notice the tighter gastric band on your stomach your eating habits improve

Around your stomach, the gastric band enhances the feelings of fullness

(S.PX3 after each of the above statements)

There is a feeling of fullness and satiety following food consumption

The idea to tighten the gastric band is for you to lose weight

The tighter gastric band also helps in managing your excessive eating and binge eating episodes

The food you eat starts to digest absorbed and metabolized very easily

The gastric band is painless even in a tightening state

You consume your food without any distress whenever you feel hungry

You are wise to notice the signs of hunger and eat only when hungry

Your body is in shape and getting a lot more in shape to let you reach towards your ideal image

(S.P after each of the above statements)

Your body alarms you when full with the help of this gastric band you hold yourself back from excessive food consumption

You are accustomed to chewing every bite of your healthy food for at least 40 seconds before you ingest

You mindfully observe the food you eat

You take few bites and you swallow only nutritious food

The food meets your body requirements and you quickly notice that the tightness of the gastric band supports you in overcoming your food addictions

You are living a happy life with a flat stomach and the healthy fat is only present in your body

(S.P after each of the above statements)

Your body contains only healthy fat

There is a huge reduction in the food portions you eat

Your food plate only carries healthy food options

You do this in addition to your eating habits

As a result, you have observed that the tightness of your stomach is the most comfortable experience as if the leaves of the tree

Imagine you are spending a wonderful holiday near a treehouse

This treehouse is located within the large trees with fresh leaves

The unexplainable peace you experience near the trees complement your gastric band tightness

You are ready to enjoy these experiences

(L.P after each of the above statements)

Explore the treehouse and feel your stomach tightness
As you closely observe the leaves thickness and variety of shapes you smell the salty air coming from the nearby seaside
The beach is cool and the water is healing
Right after you listen to the waves of the sea
Imagine the touch of your stomach as a flat, slim and ideal figure
The wooden barks are rough like the rocky road but the visual sensations in your mind are enchanting
This place has a wide range of treats for you
(M.PX2 after each of the above statements)

Dig your feet into the warm soil, which is clear and clean
The earthlike taste is in your mouth that you are aware of
Collect all these relaxation-inducing experiences and appreciate the tightness of the gastric band around your belly
Once again with the sensory enrichment of the place you visualize
Bring yourself back to your environment from the core of your stomach
Following the counting from ten to one
You will be again present on your most comfortable piece of furniture
Ten
Nine
Eight
Seven
Six

Five
Four
Three
Two
One
Let the texture of your skin allows you to breathe in and breathe out deeply for three seconds
One
Two
Three
As you try to open your eyes feel the moments you cherish in the middle of the forests
You are back with more power and attention than before
You may sound more committed to your transformation whenever you speak
You must communicate and share the message of healing with others
Compassion is one of the best sources to get back what you want
Surround yourself with beautiful relationships and those who encourage you
Celebrate even the smallest milestones and assemble the shadows of blessings while let go of those that don't allure
(S.P after each of the above statements)

7. Do the mindful eating

Be comfortable in whatever position you are
Find a place where you can rest and lay down for a while
Focus on my voice as if there is no other voice coming into your ears
Feel the light and soft air around you
Close your eyes as if there is nothing to see
Wherever you are trying to keep your back and neck completely straight
Let your feet straight and loose
Let your palms straight and loose
Let your back straight
Focus on your hands, feet and backbone
Make sure they are all straight, loose and relaxed
(S.P after each of the above statements)

In whatever state you are in just observe
Avoid judgment but simply observe
When you complete observing you will be participating in your sensory experiencing and describing
So observe your weight on the floor or sofa on which you are resting
Observe your body from head to toe
Observe your sensations in your head
Observe your sensations in your forehead
Observe your sensations in your eyes
Observe your sensations around your nasal passage
Observe your sensations in your upper lips area

Observe your sensations in your chin and below
your lips
Observe the sensations around your lips and ears
(S.P after each of the above statements)

In whatever state you are in just observe
Avoid judgment but simply observe
When you complete observing you will be
participating in your sensory experiencing and
describing
So observe your weight on the floor or sofa on
which you are resting once again and now
Observe your neck area
Observe your sensations in your shoulders both
right and left
Observe your sensations in your arms both right
and left
Observe your sensations in your hands
Observe your sensations around your all ten fingers
of both hands
Observe your sensations in your chest
Observe your sensations in your abdomen and hips
Observe the sensations around your legs, knees,
ankles and feet till toes completely
(S.P after each of the above statements)

Completely allow yourself to reflect on your
observations
Say a word about your scan of your head area
Say a word about the scan of your forehead
Say a word about the scan of your pair of eyes
Say a word about the scan of your nose

Say a word about the scan of your upper lips and lips

Say a word about the scan of your chin and the area under the chin

Say a word about the scan of your ears

Can you completely feel the sensations without any judgments like good or bad?

Be neutral in your description of sensations and say to yourself that you let go of judgments

Affirm, "I let go of judgments about myself and others or my food and body"

(S.P after each of the above statements)

Try again and completely allow yourself to reflect on your observations again

Say a word about your scan of your area around your neck

Say a word about the scan of your shoulders

Say a word about the scan of your arms and hands, fingers and stomach

Say a word about the scan of your chest and hips

Say a word about the scan of your legs and knees

Say a word about the scan of your knees and feet

Say a word about the scan of your toes

Can you completely feel the sensations without any judgments like good or bad?

Be neutral in your description of sensations and say to yourself that you let go of judgments

Affirm, "I let go of judgments about myself and others or my food and body"

(S.P after each of the above statements)

As you let go of your judgmental attitude and beliefs
You are welcome to go deeper and deeper in your reflection of the eating process
Feel as if there is a slide in front of you
The slide is colourful like a rainbow spread across your feet
The slide invites you to giggle
Imagine you are going down nicely and enjoying the slide that has led you into a house of flowers
(S.P after each of the above statements)

The house of flowers is an excellent place to master the skill of mindful eating
That is a habit to fully experience the food consumption process with the use of five senses completely
Pay attention with an open mind as if you have picked a free and fresh flower in your right hand
The flower is of your choice
The petals are very soft
The smell is exotic
The taste of the petal when you chew from your front teeth it is soothing
The blowing of the petals with cold air is an appealing view
(S.P after each of the above statements)

The flower is very beautiful you can observe the colours in it
You can describe the type of the flower, orchid maybe, sunflower, jasmine, lily and rose or any of your choice

The texture of the flower is shown differently in different parts to you like stem, centre, petals can be different

The smell may be stronger at certain parts of the flower

The taste may be better, sweet or tangy because the flower is edible and of good quality

(S.P after each of the above statements)

Eating mindfully means to eat with complete observation

Taking part in describing the sensory characteristics of the food you eat

This process includes eating appropriately based on the needs of the body

Just right in the amount, your body needs nutrients

Eat mindfully and you observe how you let go of any distractions and emotional burdens when you eat mindfully

This source of eating makes you healthier and wiser as you pick something to eat

Choose any food of your choice to practice the mindful eating

Make sure the food is healthy and something that you eat regularly or with more ease than the other options

(S.P after each of the above statements)

Overcoming challenges in healthy eating like addictive behaviours binge eating and excessive eating are all managed with the help of mindful eating

Mindful eating allows you to eat in small bites, slowly and chewing well to digest properly so that the absorption provides you maximum nutrition from the foods with highly nutritive values
(S.P after each of the above statements)

Let's get started with the mindful eating experience of food of your choice simply by flowing the experience you had with the flower of your choice in this house of flowers
Remember to fully experience your food consumption with the use of your five senses completely
Allow yourself to hold any seasonal and fresh fruit or vegetable in your right hand
The food is of your choice
The skin and peel of the food you hold in your right hand are very soft
The smell is exotic and the food is properly washed, clean and dry
The taste of the food when you take a bite from your front teeth is soothing
The bite taking from your teeth and chewing sound in between your jaw is exciting to hear
(S.P after each of the above statements)

The food you are holding in your hand is very appealing you can observe the colours in it and acknowledge that they are attractive
You can describe the form and shape of the food, long, short, round, small or big, large or any of your choice

The texture of the food that feels to you can be different like fluffy, mushy or pulpy, hard or coarse
The smell may be stronger, sweet or citric
The taste may be delicious, your taste buds enjoy it as the ripped and grown product of nature
(S.P after each of the above statements)

Take the best use of your imagination to observe the appearance of the food
Notice the colours, how many colours are there? Which ones? What are these colours? Are they darker? Light or pale or bright? Are there any lines on the food that you can observe? Any depths or any pressure?
As you have observed that now how do you describe, participate in a word that how is the food visually and what it means to you without any judgments
Take your time and describe for few seconds
1
2
3
4
5
Hope you are done
Now we can proceed further with the sensory experience of the food
(S.P after each of the above statements)

Take the best use of your imagination to observe the sound of the food when you eat
Take a small and gentle bite

Notice the bite as you get the tiny little portion of the food in your mouth

First, it touches your lips then you grab it tightly between the lips and pass it on to the teeth

That bite sound is unique and you take the bite in then chew and the whole jaw with tongue mixed in saliva churns down the food

As you have observed that now how do you describe, participate in a word that how is the food eating voices and what it means to you without any judgments

Take your time and describe for few seconds

1

2

3

4

5

Hope you are done

Now we can proceed further with the sensory experience of the food

(S.P after each of the above statements)

Take the best use of your imagination to observe the texture of the food when you touch and taste

How your skin on the hands feels the food when it comes in contact with it

Take a small and gentle bite again

Notice the feeling on your lips as you take a bite and the tiny little portion of the food in your mouth is mixed with a whole new process

First, it touches your lips it may give a soothing and pleasant sensation then you grab it tightly between the lips and pass it on to the teeth then this gives another texture of the food as you cut it down and try to tear to ingest

As you have observed that now how do you describe, participate in a word that how is the food eating textures that you felt and what it means to you without any judgments

Take your time and describe for few seconds

1

2

3

4

5

Hope you are done

Now we can proceed further with the sensory experience of the food

(S.P after each of the above statements)

Take the best use of your imagination one more time to observe the aroma and taste of the food when you touch and chew

How your nose finds the smell and feels the food when it comes in contact with it

Take a small and gentle bite again

Notice the original taste of the food and the juicy mouth secretions

As you have observed that now how do you describe, participate in a word that how is the food aroma and flavour that you experienced and what it means to you without any judgments

Take your time and describe for few seconds

1

2

3

4
5
Hope you are done
(S.P after each of the above statements)

As you have done very well in the practice of mindful eating
Affirm, "I am committed to eating mindfully whenever I eat and I accept that it is very helpful in managing my weight and keeping me slimmer, leaner and smarter"
Feel as if there is a staircase fully covered with flowers above your head like a crown to pass under it in front of you
The stairs are very bright and colourful like a rainbow spread across your feet
The slide invites you to giggle and takes you back into deep relaxation from the depths of your mindfully eating attitude
Imagine you are waking up from a dream with a new eating habit very nicely and cheerfully crossing below the shade of flowers from the house of the flowers
(S.P after each of the above statements)

Again, take your focus back on your body
Observe how you feel at your straight and loose feet
Observe how you feel at your straight and loose palms
Focus on your hands, feet and backbone
Make sure they are all straight, loose and relaxed again

Open your eyes as if there is relaxation everywhere
Feel comfortable in whatever position you are
Observe your entire place around you where you
are resting at the moment
Focus on any voice that is coming into your ears
Feel the light and soft air around you
Enjoy healthy eating from today a lot more
(S.P after each of the above statements)

8. Improving body image, gaining more confidence and combating social anxieties

Close your eyes
Softly and gently
Let your head find a support
A soft and holding support that makes your neck straight and at ease
This is the time to receive something in your life for your health and wellness
To begin receiving join your hands and open them like a book
Nice, now hold the hands in this position facing your palms towards the ceiling
As you do this place the back of your hands on your stomach and imagine the gift is coming downward
Let's open the gift gradually
(M.PX3 after each of the above statements)

Own your gift and unwrap it
This is exciting and the procedure of unwrapping may be stimulating just like you experience any anxieties throughout the day
During your anxiety, the signs may be heart throbbing, sweaty hands, jerking and shaking, loss of energy and headache
Such experience might be an indicator of the fear of evaluation that emerges from the criticisms of other people about your body posture, physique and weight
A flabby stomach can be the reason or double chin

It is possible that some people are critical and some are just ignorant of the factors involved in this condition

There are our beliefs involved in the development of anxiety

The social anxiety that specifically appears in a social situation is related to the myths and assumptions that people don't like overweight bodies or they want to see only slim bodies

Such assumptions and myths are coped with with the help of helpful affirmations

These positive affirmations must be recalled daily

Affirm now "I have the ability and skills to achieve my goals for healthy eating and healthy weight without any fear of what people think of my body"

Now take a slow deep breath, inhale and exhale

Continue affirming with my voice and stay focused

I am free of any worry that people are watching me

I stay comfortable whatever the situation is

I do not worry about letting people watch me because I look beautiful and healthy

I stop worry whenever I step out of my room

I want to get freedom from my worries

I am beginning to overcome the anxiety and I learn to stay calm and peaceful

I relax whenever I get a chance to take a deep breath and I usually show compassion to myself by counting my deep breaths

A little progress in your condition each day is a blessing

Pay close attention to the state of your body and mind when it relaxes following the counting

The relaxation offers to you a healthy state of body and well mind
One at a time rule is the best way to get rid of workload and extra stress, pain or muscle tension
Do only one task at a time
Affirm "I am focused on my goal of mindful eating whenever I eat I quit all other tasks because the best taste is the feeling of being healthy"
As you learn to overcome the monsters of anxiety that were previously haunting you
The unwrapping of the gift is now becoming more pleasurable and slow with keen observation to take a look without any hurry or impulsivity
(M.PX3 after each of the above statements)

Listen carefully
Your body has allowed you to change the treatment you give to your body
Appreciate every inch of your body that has been transforming since the last few minutes
Your body deserved to be loved without any conditions and boundlessness
Affirm, "I love my body very much and I love my body with the treatment it deserves, I like every inch of my body and I am kind towards it all the time. Whenever I eat, I always notice how my body feels. This is an amazing feeling to be in love with my body. When I do something for my body I take care of its needs I feel better than before. My appearance is not what defines me, I am beyond the body, I am a soul and a kind heart I am compassionate and I am likeable, I survive as much life as possible and I am the whole new change that

I work for every day. As a person, my body is unique and different from anyone else in this world. This is a gift a priceless gift to me"

Let another affirmation about body image influence your mind with great pleasure

Say with me and repeat "I honour my body as a sacred place where I can pray and charity, where I can show gratitude and love, where there is no such thing like negativity and associated words"

The body is a complete world for those who live in it but the real happiness is to live with it and to live for it

Imagine sending love and kindness to every cell of your body

To all the blood running in your bloodstreams

To all the fluids within

To all the organs functioning

To all the hormones and secretions that are own temple

Silently observe each of your body existing parts internally and externally to show thankfulness and loads of appreciation

You are now completely under the spell of your existence

Affirm "I open my heart to the beautiful and kind words that I use for myself, I say positive words for my body and I only appreciate how it functions, It is a blessing and I am grateful"

Notice how a spark of energy flows within you when you say nice and strongly positive words about yourself

This is the most precious gift that you offer to yourself and your body

The body image is the perception that a human being holds for self

The size and shape doesn't define self, only the perception of self matters

There is no one else who can do this for you

Only you know about yourself the best

Be the potential for your body-image

Be the world of your mind

Affirm "I have the best image of my body in my mind, I am carefree of the perceptions of anyone else, I know my body best and this is all that matters to me for a happy and satisfying life"

There is peace within me everywhere

I allow changes in my daily routine

I allow changes in my daily food

I allow changes in my daily meals

I allow changes in my activities

I allow changes in my thoughts, as they are more flexible now

I allow changes in my emotions as I can manage them wisely

I allow changes in my self-control as it is improved

I allow changes in my letting go attitude and I am more easily letting out the doubts, regrets and complains

I only allow my perception to define myself and my perception of my body is like a gift that I am receiving

I am opening the gift and this is my self that is sparkling, attractive and productive

This gift has to enlighten my mind and soul

My body is being praised and cared for with this gift

This is the outcome of this gift that I am holding that I love my body
(M.PX3 after each of the above statements)

Affirm, " I believe that I am getting more and more confident every day without any effort or distress"
I have the talent to express my thoughts politely towards myself
I am quite clever and clear in my mind about my confidence
I am aware of the wonderful functioning of my mind and body
I have vocabulary and fluency in my speech that has the power to influence my opinions
I am a good communicator to express my expression of admiration towards myself
I am a very confident person and an attractive soul
I love my personality traits as well like I deeply love my body
My love and likeness for my body and mind getting deeper and deeper and this is bringing me closer and closer to myself and my relationship with a healthy lifestyle is getting stronger and stronger
With this deep connection, the vibes of my motivation are spreading all around my body and my cells are all covered with the light, glow and joy of a healthy mind
This is the expression of deep and permanent confidence that is flowing within me
Anyone can witness the beauty of this confidence in my expression and communication, my physical movements, gestures and facial expressions

I feel so connected with my mind and the functioning of my body

As a spiritual being, I am open to the future gifts and blessings of the universe that are meant to reach my soul

This has been the awakening of my overall self and I exist to a wide array of positivity and beneficial range of world where my thoughts linger in search of even more confidence myself

Everything around me is spun like a silky threat of smiles

I am getting more and more relaxed and more and more confident as I realize that I am feeling very happy and grateful

Achieving confidence is a step of personal success as a vital sign to approach more opportunities

I am getting more and more confident as the days are passing

This is very special to me that this experience is multi-dimensional

I am honestly being in love with my beautiful and confident body like a vase that I bring to my room and place that at a higher place away from any hazards

That vase is the eye candy for everyone and the colours are very calming

This calming effect is my choice and I prefer everything in my life and for my health that is calming

Now let's get prepared for another part of this gift that you are holding in your hands, 1, 2, and 3

(M.PX3 after each of the above statements)

Remind yourself that "I let go of any addictions that didn't serve me ever because I am mentally strong and I know the importance of eating healthy and pure foods from the blessings of nature, I understand that the food I eat can cover only a small area in my stomach is the size of my fist and I manage to measure my meal based on my fist size. On my plate, I always add a portion of fresh sliced or chopped coleslaw and greens, one portion of beans and only one portion from whole grains and lean meat"

As you find yourself vulnerable to falling into a loop of temptations and cravings for unhealthy food

There is always an option to enjoy a cheat meal, once in seven days or more

The food addiction or obsession with food is now resolved from within

I am pure and clean and feel sober like a new child

A new baby like steps I would like to take to hold the gift in my hand that I unwrapped

It is just as beautiful as the soft and tint of the skin a baby has

The gift is my health and wellness that is full of confidence, more and more confidence with an admiring body image

The gift supplied me with a life with clarity

The anxieties vanish and the addictive behaviours are gone away

The storms of the emotions and thunders of my stomach hunger pangs due to dieting or distress following excessive eating are now flowing like an obedient light that glows and glows spreading the hope all around my body and my skin reflects the glow from the light of hope

Affirm, "I feel as confidant as I am master my eating habits with self-control and wisdom"

(M.PX3 after each of the above statements)

Open your eyes

Softly and gently

Let your head turn right and then left

This is the time to say thank you openly and express gratitude for the gift of your health and wellness

To begin this expression join your hands together and close them like a book

Nice, now hold the hands in this position facing your palms towards each other and bow down your head a bit

As you do this gesture the outcome is the assurance that gifts stay with you forever

Let's take a deep breath showing gratitude to the universe

(M.PX3 after each of the above statements)

9. Removal of the gastric band

Get deeply relax
Imagine a shiny glass staircase is present in front of you
As you get more and more relaxed and comfortable at your place you will be able to move ahead smoothly
The footsteps that you will take might lead you to the lovely transformation of your body
You reach a newer version of yourself and your deep down desires may appear fulfilled
Desires about your body image and lesser fat, slimmer tummy and leaner you
You are going to witness your transformation today after few minutes
You might feel joy at your peak
(M.PX3 after each of the above statements)

Leave your body completely loose
Image your closeness to your created body as an outcome of the gastric band placement and tightening for the past few days
The wish of your soul is approaching completion
Starting a healthier life is an art that you have mastered
You have mastered this skill and now you are competent to eat healthy food and continue a slimmer life
Major changes in the past few days have dropped your weight to a remarkable level

With the help of the gastric band, your belly seems slimmer and smarter
Around your stomach, the skin glows and it feels tight with a complete youth
(S.PX4 after each of the above statements)

Take a deep nice breath again
Breathe in and out from the depths of your stomach
Let your body move according to your nasal passage contraction and relaxation
Your lungs take in the air and your mouth blows out the air in a pattern that you are watching regularly
Inhale as much as possible to the fullest capacity of your lungs
Let the lungs spread like a balloon and watch them rise for a few seconds, 1, 2, 3
Now continue focusing the system to exhale the air out for a few seconds, 1, 2, 3
(S.P after each of the above statements)

Very good, close your eyes tightly and imagine the staircase made of beautiful shining glass
The glass looks crystal clear, clean and transparent
You can see through the glass there are metal bars to support the stairs
The stairs are firm and glorious
The view is mind-blowing and for the next 10 seconds you will be moving downward using this staircase
As I count begin stepping on the first stair
1
Move to the next stair

2
Continue
3
Keep going
4
5
6
7
8
9
10
There is complete peace all around you
(S.P after each of the above statements)

Pay attention to where this staircase takes you
It is your favourite place
The same area where you took the initiative of this
gastric band that has changed your lifestyle
Enjoy this feeling of accomplishment
Allow yourself to attract more and more blessings
other than the desirable body weight and shape that
the gastric band has given you
You have been offered to secure this achievement
for the future
Throughout life, the slimmer and leaner belly stays
with you
Without any doubt, you know this better than
positivity transforms attitude towards food and our
body
Your support to your body is the overall result of
your gastric band

Your confidence, willpower, trust and
determination has brought up this moment of
success
Focus on the outcome of your body
There is a flat stomach and healthy-looking skin
(L.P after each of the above statements)

A healthy-looking feeling that you have is
associated with your sensations of the gastric band
effectiveness
It is easier for you now to keep moving with the
same routine and lesser amount of food
You buy, choose, pick and prepare only nutritious
and delicious food
Your experience with the gastric band is simply
natural
This relationship has built because you have
achieved the goals you settled at the beginning
Watch your radiance with the power of your mind
Your skin is smooth and supple
You are smaller in body size
You are in love with what you do
Visibly the vibes are your reality
(M.P after each of the above statements)

You feel your days are much more balanced similar
to the food on the plate that you eat
Your amazing skill of choices and changes that you
adopted for your health is appreciated
Your style of cooking and methods to mindfully get
in touch with your food is a great progress
Your complete existence has shown a pretty smile
Listen to this your body is saying you thank you

Imagine the colour of your gastric band around your stomach

Place your hand on it and feel the band is of your favourite colour

The most suitable thickness and smallness of the gastric band compliments your tiny waistline

You can proudly say that you can keep this flat stomach daily in maintenance with your time and dedication towards a healthy lifestyle

The recommendations for your healthy eating are simple, quick and beneficial

You completely learn and educate yourself with the application process of the brave and bold task for eating healthy

(S.P after each of the above statements)

You are gratefully in love with the function of the gastric band that has now been completed successfully

You must proceed with the removal of the gastric band

For this purpose, you commit to your desired body weight and image that you would control your food amounts and calorie intake whenever you intend to consume a meal

You accept and agree with the free choice of eating healthy effortlessly and allow the removal of gastric band

Following this path to freedom and commitment simultaneously, every moment is a witness of your dedication to yourself

You share this genuine experience and feelings
attached to the freedom from the burdens of your
body
Imagine a vast limitless sight of the lake you know
about
Next, the courage is going to increase without even
the gastric band on your stomach
Your skin of the belly is smarter and lighter
(S.P after each of the above statements)

As the gastric band removes the skin becomes more
sensitive to the air
Feel fresh as soon as the gastric band removes
The lightness of your belly might sound like a
feather flying over the vast limitless lake
The responsible attitude of carrying the gastric band
is shifting to the easiest commitment of maintaining
healthy eating habits for a healthy body and mind
Your motivation strikes up as you make up your
mind to create a big difference without the aid of
the gastric band
Unlike the presence of a gastric band, you are
capable to try creative ideas that lit up your
intuition for improvement in overall health
The energy that you have gained is getting shinier
and shinier
You have spread the light in the universe around
you
Your shine vibrates and resonates with the skies
Your ability to forgive all those who ever criticize
your body is getting flared up
The tendency to forgive yourself and others show
that your tenderness and love is above all

You are talented enough to manifest your dreams into truth

The undeniable truth is that you eat as your body needs without the gastric band

(L.P after each of the above statements)

At a very slow pace

Show compassion to self and blow kisses to others in your imagination

You feel more and more relaxed

The deeply and deeply relaxed posture of yours like you to lose your muscles

As all the parts of your body relax the gastric band loses up as well

The gastric band is loosening for few seconds

1

2

3

4

5

6

7

Observe the motion of the gastric band

It's just slipping away from your skin

The soft procedure of the gastric band removal is painless and soundless

The only voice you hear for the next few seconds is of your peaceful deep breathing

1

2

3

Such a happy event has happened

(S.P after each of the above statements)

This happens due to what you like
Your preference has been strengthened for fresh
ingredients like whole grains
The foods that all contain high nutritive value is
your only preference to consume daily
Your stomach fills fast when you eat a smaller
portion of food
You eat short meals and you nourish your body
with lightweight naturally made snacks
(S.P after each of the above statements)

Imagine you love to chew corns for minutes
Boiled warm corns covered in herbs, chillies and
lemon
This stimulates the smell of tangy flavours
The crunch and crisp is an essential part of your
meal
The food equals the size of your fist and you feel
full whenever you eat that food only in hunger
The foods you consume with minimum sugar
intake, minimum fat content and minimum salt are
the best for your mind and soul
Your body feels rested when you eat food at room
temperature
You must facilitate your body with refreshing and
metabolism-boosting beverages free of soda and
artificial tasting
Our body reciprocates us
What we offer we get back
Give your body soul-enriching food
Drink mind and lemon
Blend yoghurt, fruits, raw veggies and honey
Drink milk and toss plain cheese on salads

Cut and slice the cucumbers, bell peppers, carrots and eggplants
Feel how you like the process of juices coming out
Smell how you get excited with the aroma
Know how you welcome the taste
See how you invite the variety
Listen to the knife on the cutting board when chopping the raw washed food helps your digestive system
As a healthy eater, the temperature of food to choose for storage and serving is all in your hands
Observe the strikes the crunchy and raw clean food make in your gums and jaw
This is so pure and it impresses your senses
(M.PX3 after each of the above statements)

Pay attention as if you look at the sky above a window in the dining room
The chair and table are of black wood
Your sight tries to catch the highest lengths of the sky where cotton balls like clouds are floating
It makes your cheeks blush and your lips going on a half-smile
Slightly spread the lips apart and murmur, "I love my body, I eat healthily, I eat clean and I eat raw, I eat in moderation"
Taking yourself back from the beautiful sightseeing's of your favourite place
Say goodbye to the generous gastric band
Look for the glass staircases that take you back from the depths of your transformation
Leaving behind the cold air, the noise of water and boats those move within

The glass staircase is not too far
(S.PX2 after each of the above statements)

Start walking and take small steps, these small steps
also help you when you walk daily
The daily walk is one of the methods to maintain
weight, to burn daily calories and to keep stomach
slimmer
Be mindful as you take these steps on the road
going to the stairs
As you observe walking steps, imagine the steady
walking to open a new chapter of your life
A healthier life full of success and happiness is
waiting for you to approach
Every morning or evening or anytime at least 30
minutes of walking can become an assurance of
your healthy weight maintenance to meet your
personal goals and to supply you with power
(M.P after each of the above statements)

Imagine the footsteps provide plenty of energy,
courage, motivation and spark to stay on your
health goals
Walk confidently, slowly; continue for few more
minutes that direct your future
For young and older, for men and women for all
ages and professionals, the walk is safe
You walk with complete comfort
As you walk, witness the comfort is flowing from
your feet
From the base of your feet, the toes, heels and sole
the comfort is on your ankles

The comfort is contagious, slow, deep and consistent
Notice the comfort pumps relaxation to the legs, above to the hips, above to your backbone and chest
It becomes more and more relaxing to walk and you can feel it in your chest and neck and shoulders and face
This is fine for you to walk for an hour and you become a regular walker within few days
(L.P after each of the above statements)

Now, look your staircase is right in your sight
The staircase is made of beautiful shining glass
The glass looks crystal clear, clean and transparent
You can see through the glass there are metal bars to support the stairs
The stairs are firm and glorious
The view is mind-blowing and for the next 10 seconds you will be moving upward using this staircase
As I count begin stepping on the tenth stair
10
Move to the next stair
9
Continue
8
Keep going
7
6
5
4
3
2

1
Open your eyes
There is complete peace all around you
(S.P after each of the above statements)

10. Continue healthy lifestyle

Find a comfortable place for you to rest
Straighten your back and limbs
Gather all the kind intentions for your body
Recall some of the smiling memories of yourself
Laugh out loud for your achievements so far
Open yourself for a new experience associated with
your body
Your body weight is lighter
Your body image is ideal
Your body is now toned
The stomach fat has burned
You see your existence with excitement
Your excitement to continue receiving blessings for
yourself remains the same
You are the witness of the shaping of your
relationship with food into a healthier one
(M.PX2 after each of the above statements)
Relax your all body parts
Focus on your body parts one by one from head to
toe
Progressively pay attention towards the relaxation
of muscles and healthy cells functioning in each
area of your body
Take a deep breath when you focus on your face
muscles
Take a deep breath when you pay attention you're
your relaxed neck and shoulders
Take a deep breath when you imagine that your
chest muscles are relaxing

Take a deeper breath as you feel that your arms;
hands, palms and fingers are relaxing
The energy is flowing from your shoulders to your
fingernails
(L.P after each of the above statements)
Take a deep breath when you focus on your belly
muscles
Take a deep breath when you pay attention you're
your relaxed thighs and legs
Take a deep breath when you imagine that your
hips and feet are relaxing
Take a deeper breath as you feel that your feet,
heels, toes and sole are relaxing
The energy is flowing from your lower back to the
end of your limbs
This progressive scan of your body muscles
refreshes your ability to focus on your
transformation
You are as much determined to maintain your body
weight as much as you are relaxed and in love with
your gastric band outcome
(S.P after each of the above statements)
Let your eyes closed slowly and naturally as you
count from one to five
With each number, tighten your closed eyes
One for your eyes closed
Two for your eyes closing with tightness
Three for your eyes closed tighter and tighter
Four to feel that your eyes are now tightening and
tightening even more
Five to leave your eyes closed as tight as possible
Coming down from your eyes to your chest
Breathing continues to relax your nerves

Pay attention to flow in and out of the air
Pay attention to the voice of your breathing
Pay attention to the texture of your skin above your lungs and stomach
(S.P after each of the above statements)
Feel the softness and smoothness of these body spots for your awareness
For three seconds just be grateful for whatever you have achieved so far
Aim to maintain and manage the achieved desirable state of body and mind
Imagine your lighter body is now capable of freely floating on a smooth and clear surface
Let your body fly in the air without any support
Imagine these sensations of touching air with your skin
Smell the air around your lighter body
Choose a colour to indicate the fluffy air surrounding your slimmer body
(S.PX3 after each of the above statements)
Allow the air to come near your ears and feel as if the clouds are spinning a web of mesh to support your body
Your hair is lighter in weight
Your head floats like a flower
Your cheeks are deeply soft and glowing
It appears that your face, your neck, upper body, lower body are all weightless
Like a cute balloon, you love this skydiving
Your muscles, cells and bones are weightless
Your stomach is lighter and smaller
At your complete resting state

You can make this position a routine for your self-discovery

Loosen your body completely once again and release all the things you usually hold

(L.PX4 after each of the above statements)

Take ten steps now from one to ten towards a new initiative of healthy eating as a lifestyle

Going down in the depths of your mind you are going to make healthy living a reality

Take step one and pay attention to the natural herbal fruits and vegetable farm downstairs

Take step two and you can smell the natural earthy smell of natural ingredients

Take step three and you can see fresh foods are ready for you to taste

Take further steps four, five and six so that you can grab the hanging fresh foods from the longer trees

At steps seven, eight and nine you can reach the herbal plants with exotic benefits

Put your feet on step ten and you can feel the raw texture of the soil

(S.P after each of the above statements)

Visit the whole farm and enjoy it

This healthy lifestyle is at the core of your mind where the belief takes rest

Leave yourself free in the middle of this farm and create beautiful memories

Associate yourself with the world's best available foods that are just grown from the earthly sources

This is the deepest place of your creative imagination

Where you learn to manifest a vast variety of raw foods and naturally made beverages

(S.P after each of the above statements)

Cherish each of the moments you stay here at this heavenly place

This farmland is limitless

The sounds you hear around you are the rustling of leaves

The soil particles are rich to enable nutritious foods to grow out

You experience freedom and you live like you have achieved all your goals related to body weight and healthy eating

Continue picking the fruits of your choice

The fruits that are fully packed with pulp and fibre

Pick the vegetables covered in soil to add to your daily meals

You have a routine to add the preparation of these naturally grown foods

(S.PX3 after each of the above statements)

You acknowledge the presence of these foods in your life

The air seems to dance and covering you all over

The smell of the fresh herbs continue

Your selection of being a part of this healthy life is aligned with your healthy life goals

You deserve appreciation for these accomplishments

You only add honey when you crave sweet

You make your sodium intake minimum per day about a pinch

You use herbal spices and lots of leaves over your salads

You eat clean and love the Mediterranean diet

106

Nuts and seeds daily enrich your smoothies and shakes

Continue nurturing yourself with these foods of great value

(S.PX2 after each of the above statements)

Make this choice of healthy food consumption a priority

Add daily walk for fast metabolism

Fast metabolism equals lesser fat storage on your belly

Prefer to chew whole grains, pulses and lentils, boiled beans and meat slices with egg

Stay with the use of cooking methods like grilling, boiling and roasting

Eat raw whereas possible

Eat till you feel full

Use hunger and fullness signals of your body in account to maintain the eating habits

Limit the intake of food when you feel full

Feel full with foods containing the higher nutritive value

(S.P after each of the above statements)

Enlist some snacks in the core of your mind and register them to use only when you crave in between meals

Limit processed foods and avoid any ready-made food consumption

Enjoy the food only in their true sense

Imagine yourself handling a handful of natural food items for each meal

The portion contains green leafy vegetables, fibre rich foods and some other varieties of your preference

Your dairy portion is necessary
Include a cup of yoghurt or milk or other dairy
made recipes in each of your daily meals
Your day become purely delicious
For breakfast sometimes boil protein sources and
sometimes mix a bowl of oats with warm milk
(M.P after each of the above statements)
Now try the addition of some crisp in your foods
The crunch of the veggies in rainbow colours
Purple, green, orange, yellow and blue
Make sure you add all in a week
Toss some corn and olives with while meat and
lean cuts they are also very healthy
The choice is yours
Only options are discussed
Serve yourself the food at a room temperature
You stay focused
Your focus is health
The snacks are your favourites
You resist all artificial flavours and colours
You resist junks
Lower down the fats, salt and sugar
Energy bars are excellent to chew
Chew till you completely enjoy the textures, juices
and smell mindfully
(L.P after each of the above statements)
Affirm " I am a healthy eater daily"
Affirm, " I am getting slimmer and slimmer, leaner
and leaner"
Affirm, "I can manage my eating and I control the
unnecessary temptations"
You know very well that healthy foods are the
secret of your weight management

Your choice of food is your fuel
For instant energy, you always eat something light
and loaded with nutrients
You drink plain water most of the time
Your daily intake of water is 10 glasses
Continue imagining the attainment of all those
foods that are in your access and good for your
mental and physical health
(S.P after each of the above statements)
As a healthy eater, you are passionate about the
preparation of food at home
The recipes are in your access
You keep the dishes simple and ingredients less
You make the food with your own hands so that
you make sure that you stick to the healthy goals
regularly
This is an easy task to know what foods are good
for health and what we can eat daily
Feel the freshness and glow on your face and skin
all over your body
You are getting lighter and lighter as you eat
Affirm, "I am getting healthier and healthier as I
follow healthy dietary habits"
As much as you are satisfied with the healthy food
choices for yourself you stay healthy
You are capable of keeping your weight in
moderation
Eat-in moderation and track your weight once a
month
Write some notes whenever you feel there are some
challenges
The answers to cope with the challenges comes
from the core of your mind

Your healthy eating practice is good for your smart, thin, pretty and flat belly

Your tummy only invites food that is according to your needs

You have the strength to take healthy steps for yourself

You feel beautiful as an outcome

(S.P after each of the above statements)

Water has become your best drink

At this farm, you explore the healthy lifestyle

The lifestyle that continues to be your preference

You enjoy whole foods and colourful natural' gifts

Clean the food that you buy to eat raw

Wash the foods properly and your hands as well

The foods with high water content are very refreshing

They have a cooling effect like the open farmland

The direct sun gives hope and happiness

The fresh air let you breathe to your fullest

The cells of your body functions multiply and replace all the time

Healthy food cleanses you and removes all the toxins

Healthy food flushes out your unrequired impurities

(S.P after each of the above statements)

The place where you are present at the moment

Imagine it with complete focus

Watch out all the sides of the land

Wherever you see you see the bliss

The sky has a blue hue above you

Clouds are floating peacefully there is calmness all around

The quietness has the appearance of the foods only

Be mindful of what you eat daily
Continue to follow the routine of healthy food choices
Pick those foods always that are natural and nutritious
Your food consumption do meet your body needs without adding an excessive burden
(S.P after each of the above statements)
This is your future your healthy routine has become your destiny
As you realize you have lived these moments completely
Begin moving towards the soil-filled staircase
The staircase is ready for you to move back upwards
As you listen to the counting ten to one flow your mind in a smooth manner
Take the first step on the tenth stair
Now one step more and you are on nine
Eight
Seven
Continue climbing
Six
Five
Four
Three
Two
One
A new morning awaits you
Get yourself out of the depths of your mind and get settled to open your eyes very very slowly
(S.P after each of the above statements)

Keep it up you do a marvellous discovery to
monitor your mind
Be in harmony with your healthy goals
This journey has remained successful all the time
Wish you satisfaction ahead
Every day and every second
You have made this choice
Your life is healthy
Eating is healthy
Shopping is healthy!
(S.P after each of the above statements)

11. Work on taking the food and eating in your control

Its time to place your hands and arms in the most comfortable position and place as you can

Its time to relax and listen to the only voice that is directly in contact with you to allow you to relax

Let this voice guides you to become more and more deeply and deeply relaxed

Let me show you that you hear this voice to direct you to a more self-control

Take your time and close your eyes whenever you feel best

In the next few moments, you would be laying down with the most peaceful and calm body

(L.P after each of the above statements)

So, in short, you are helping yourself with following this voice

As you continue listening silently and without any other sound your breathing comes to your awareness

Breathing is a beautiful phenomenon and it flows naturally in a continuous rhythm

As you might have an idea that breathing is not in our awareness because we stay busy and keep our minds involved in many other things but today let yourself be aware of your breathing

Breathe fully, freely, deeply as much as you can

For the next few seconds practice this without any judgment

Let your nasal sounds speak
(L.P after each of the above statements)

Prepare yourself for alternate nostril breathing
This is one of the most soothing ways to treat you
with kindness
The kindest act that we ever do is to let go of all the
pain and stress so that we can sleep and rest
restfully
Take your right hand to your nose and with the help
of the index finger press the right nostril to inhale
from the left nostril
Now, leave and shift your finger to press the left
nostril and exhale from the right nostril
I believe you are a quick and smart learner, let's
repeat once again
Take your right hand to your nose and with the help
of the index finger press the right nostril to inhale
from the left nostril
Now, leave shift your finger to press the left nostril
and exhale from the right nostril
Great, time to take your left hand to your nose and
with the help of the index finger press the left
nostril to inhale from the right nostril
Now, leave and shift your finger to press the right
nostril and exhale from the left nostril
I believe you are a quick and smart learner, let's
repeat once again
Great, time to take your left hand to your nose and
with the help of the index finger press the left
nostril to inhale from the right nostril
Now, leave and shift your finger to press the right
nostril and exhale from the left nostril

(S.P after each of the above statements)

By doing this practice, you can switch your body
and mind to a relaxed state whenever and wherever
you can
Relaxation is a priority and key to maintaining a
behaviour
There may be 100's of voices that you hear daily
but the only voice that matters is the voice of your
soul
The inner voice is the most reliable, the
trustworthy, and the most melodious
(M.P after each of the above statements)
In the depths of your soul, there is a place where
self-control is activated
Get down in the depths of your soul
Imagine there is a staircase leading you to the
unknown secrets of your self-control activation
With my voice imagine the movement of your feet
going down straight to the depth of your soul from
As I count from 1-10, imagine going downstairs
keeping your attention in the middle of your chest
where your heart is beating
1, 2, 3, 4, 5, 6, 7, 8, 9, 10 (S.P between each)
Now you are at the depth of your soul and a cool
blue, peaceful light ball is in front of you
Continue to breathe deeply; the light ball is your
self-control, ready to take in your hands
(M.P after each of the above statements)

As you relax, imagine a picture in your mind where
you idealize your personality as a person who is an
example of the best self-control

Self-control is strength, there is strength in the control that you take on yourself, on your obsessions about excessive eating, on your emotions letting you eat without any need and self-control is also your mood to monitor your food intake and to remind yourself that it is important to abide by the commitment of healthy eating, slimmer stomach and leaner fat-free body for the rest of your life
(L.PX2 after each of the above statements)

Focus on purpose is the foremost condition of self-control
Most of the impulsive decisions and actions we take under the influence of our irrational thoughts and negative emotions are not related to our food intake and also have no relation to the appetite
Let the purpose be your sole guide to empower you to seek, ask and practice self-control without any force and external pressures
Shed out all those moments from your memory when someone else actions and comments made you lose your self-control
You are intelligent and you direct your significant journey of maintaining a healthier weight, slimmer body shape and glowing skin with the help of self-control while you consume food and drink water
(M.P after each of the above statements)

Beating temptations is another milestone for self-control
One way to beat temptations is consistency with discipline

116

Eating and drinking on a fixed schedule can help
It can be flexible based on your feasibility and
routine
Do what matches your life and develop a higher
character of self-control
Step up in your power of seeking self-control and
practising it whenever you mindlessly linger your
eyes on unhealthy food
Be mindful of the triggers and choose an action to
cope with it
(L.P after each of the above statements)

Overcome the unpredictable actions by planning
eating time and foods with appropriate quantity in
advance
This is the quality that you add to your eating habits
There are many faces of self-control that you learn
here
The moment you decide to take hold your
conscience helps you
There is no need to talk to anyone, do a private
speech meditation of few seconds for the support
Just try it right now, pick a word for your ease to
verbalize when you are in the need of self-control
It may be bind, it may be fixed or comes back
After you choose, repeat your selected word five
times
Now count your fingers of the right hand
Now count your fingers on the left hand
Wow! You just delayed your gratification for the
whole 15 seconds
This is what you need whenever you need self-
control

A break and pause of 15 seconds is shown to
release the momentary temptation
Just look away from the temptation for 15 seconds
Stay as far away as you can where there is no
aroma of the temptation
This is the formula to your willpower too
(M.P after each of the above statements)

Another self-control tactic is improving stamina
with the help of daily movements
The movements need to be easy
Quick and short
You can move your body as you want
Try Zumba, join a dance class, go on a walk with a
friend or shake your body with the help of a song
alone
(M.P after each of the above statements)
Whenever you move your body and stretch a bit
you realize it is supplying even more brightness and
colour to your blue self-control ball with power,
patience and delayed action
Affirm with your body movement "I move my body
and experience self-control"
(M.P after each of the above statements)

Other pleasurable activities might help you as well
Keep an activity diary with you wherever you go
Include a list of 10 exciting mind-diverting
activities that give you self-control to maintain your
focus on self-control over food
Something that stops your cravings

Read a joke, share a quote, write something interesting, take a photo and delete it, these tasks are at no cost but saves you 100's calories
Always take a big water bottle in your bag and drink 10 cups per day
Water manages weight and cravings before appetite signals as well
Only eat when the empty stomach and enjoy life lightly
(M.P after each of the above statements)

Look for what's in your plate that contains protein and much of it to cover the unnecessary fats and sugar that leads to excessive eating
Skip the alcoholic beverages and cut down the packaged juices
With these tips, you would see a visible difference in your ability to manage your trend towards eating unhealthy foods to a great extent
There is sufficient research evidence to convince someone
When you distance yourself from food within meal gaps and outside fixed schedule for meals you can drop down the harm from 50-60%
(M.P after each of the above statements)

Maintain energy levels
Let me explain another secret to managing self-control when food is present around you and there is no appetite for that food exist in your body
Always chew some energy bars, take a zip-lock bag with fruit, dates or nuts to avoid extreme hunger pangs for a longer time

As you stay away from food somewhat fill your stomach so that you usually don't get back to food without boundaries when available

The body needs food on time to prevent the excessive storage of food following longer times of empty stomach

Maintain a reciprocal relationship with your body and mind

Let them take care of you in exchange for providing them with care

(M.P after each of the above statements)

Build associations between the work and relaxation by connecting them with stress-busting activities

Stress anchors excessive eating and stress management means no cravings and less eating

It is always a great idea to connect your stress with a healthy food bite

Take an example of spinach, equals to the size of your smallest finger, chew it for at least 60 seconds

Observe and describe the taste, smell, colour and texture

Listen to the jaws churning up and juices of your saliva getting mixed with it

All the stress vanishes away and for few seconds you find a soothing trick for your nerves

(M.P after each of the above statements)

Review upon the self-control methods you have learned today

The understanding of these methods gives you more and more deep insight about using them

Be flexible and find several different ways to soothe you daily so that the mind stays relaxed as the relaxed mind keeps control of the actions and act logically for a health-oriented lifestyle
Take proper sleep and make a proper meal plan
Review your plan weekly and make adjustments whereas necessary to cope up with the circumstantial changes and unavoidable life challenges
(M.P after each of the above statements)

Observe deeply the blue light ball that is present in your hands
You are taking it back with you out of your soul
The activation of the blue light ball has been done as you progressively learn the tactics to practice self-control
The ball is very powerful and you can always take it in your hands with closed eyes whenever you lose control and search for something to get back to self-control
(M.P after each of the above statements)

The same staircase is going upward in the form of 10 stairs (S.P)
You may climb up towards the external world, one at a time, slowly and with peace 1, 2, 3, 4, 5, 6, 7, 8, 9, and 10 (S.P between each number)
Deep breathe as you are out of that staircase with the blue light ball of self-control in your hands that you have gained well now

You have reached the place from where we moved ahead to the glorious success of achieving your health-related goals

Open your eyes to the physical objects that are present around you as you have formed required habits and self-control is now your strength
(M.P after each of the above statements)

Conclusion

Hypnosis is a science and so does the weight loss and associated biochemical or psychosocial processes. The benefits of using hypnosis for weight loss are numerous. The first and foremost effect of using hypnosis is deep relaxation. Then there comes the formation of the habit for healthy eating, picking nutritious food without compromising delicious tastes and flavours. For some people, all these changes come slowly than others. The rate of change may be related to the willingness and motivation that the person shows who follow this method of healing eating problems. Hypnosis works for all different when it comes to weight loss.

Weight loss isn't any magic trick; there is no magic wand to spread a chant for a healthy eating lifestyle. There is sufficient evidence to plan diets and follow foods to avoid list for fat burn and weight management but there is no guarantee that a person is motivated and willing enough to comply with the given instructions on a piece of paper unless someone deliberately believes that the diet would help them. Weight loss is not only a matter of self-control but also a way to feel happiness and satisfaction. An ideal weight elicits the self-image in a person's mind to support further performance in one's occupational and personal life. We continue eating the ideal way possibly and automatically. Weight loss is not the only benefit with the help of gastric band hypnosis. Other benefits are overcoming emotional eating, dealing with malnutrition, getting rid of the foods that are harmful to human beings, improving self-image and nutritious eating habits development. There are many more psychological and social benefits that individuals may experience with time. The outcomes frequency and benefits differ from individual to individual because everyone is unique. Gastric band hypnosis is a useful tool that is even more powerful than the already observed. This is usually the beginning of lifetime learning with a purposeful plan with documented literature.

Weight loss is a proven outcome of hypnosis and related techniques that we associate and use with this method. Most commonly the notable results are specific to some people's contexts. Studies have shown that those who are more responsive to the hypnosis effect are compassionate, open to new experiences and selfless lovers. Personality traits play a role in the ease of the change process. On the other hand, the more susceptible people to hypnosis are below 18 or above 40. Within gender differences, females are more drawn to hypnosis than males.
On the other hand, people are more likely to be hypnotized if the hypnotist voice and way of communication is well-practised, according to the client needs and he or she guides appropriately. Change and weight loss are the processes. That is why; we use an integrative approach to maximize the outcome and optimal human pleasure without compromising the food or abiding by any tiring

routine. Another component added to the series of this book is maintaining weight after required loss and fat burning sessions to take the most advantage of hypnosis for this purpose. Good Luck!

Reference Resource Links

1. https://www.jqph.org/index.php/JQPH/article/view/150
2. https://www.sciencedirect.com/science/article/abs/pii/S1130862119301159
3. https://link.springer.com/chapter/10.1007/978-1-4939-9098-6_17
4. http://www.ijnhs.net/index.php/ijnhs/article/view/317
5. https://www.sciencedirect.com/science/article/abs/pii/S0169260715304399
6. https://search.proquest.com/openview/f3bba7b5d087324407284cee65ee84fe/1?pq-origsite=gscholar&cbl=3912278
7. https://www.tandfonline.com/doi/abs/10.1080/08964289.2020.1842316
8. https://www.tandfonline.com/doi/abs/10.1080/00207144.2017.1314740
9. https://onlinelibrary.wiley.com/doi/abs/10.1002/acp.3730
10. https://www.intechopen.com/books/hypnotherapy-and-hypnosis/hypnosis-and-hypnotherapy-emerging-of-science-based-hypnosis
11. https://www.tandfonline.com/doi/abs/10.1080/00029157.2017.1316233
12. https://www.tandfonline.com/doi/abs/10.1080/00029157.2018.1489777
13. https://www.liebertpub.com/doi/abs/10.1089/acm.2020.0104

14. https://www.tandfonline.com/doi/abs/10.1080/0002
    9157.2016.1261678
15. https://www.emerald.com/insight/content/doi/10.11
    08/JOE-07-2019-0029/full/html
16. https://onlinelibrary.wiley.com/doi/abs/10.1111/obr
    .13003
17. https://www.tandfonline.com/doi/abs/10.1080/0020
    7144.2019.1613863
18. https://iris.unito.it/handle/2318/1633448#.YHVRp2
    hRXUo
19. https://ijbmc.org/index.php/ijbmc/article/view/174
20. https://search.proquest.com/openview/d75a70ca3c6
    9b5537a40ffe7dd856030/1?pq-
    origsite=gscholar&cbl=1896353
21. https://onlinelibrary.wiley.com/doi/abs/10.1002/978
    1119057840.ch159
22. https://psycnet.apa.org/record/2018-03961-001
23. https://onlinelibrary.wiley.com/doi/abs/10.1002/oby
    .22262
24. https://www.sciencedirect.com/science/article/abs/p
    ii/S1879729620301496

CPSIA information can be obtained
at www.ICGtesting.com
Printed in the USA
LVHW080807010621
689024LV00020B/1874